Ménière's Disease Explained

P.J. Haybach

Haybach
Hawaii, U.S.

ISBN-13:978-1979081146
ISBN-10:197908114X

Printed by Createspace

AUTHORS NOTE

This year marks the 25th year I have been studying and writing about vestibular disorders. During this time there have been many exciting developments in the field.

- Development of a relatively easy treatment for BPPV (benign paroxysmal positional vertigo).

- Discovery of dehiscence of the superior semicircular canal.

- Development of vestibular evoked myogenic potential (VEMP) testing.

- Identification of migraine as a causer of vestibular symptoms.

- Injection of drugs into the middle ear from where they enter the inner ear.

- Bedside tests of eye movement

Despite many advances, Ménière's disease continues to be a hard nut to crack, in part because the most basic information about the structure and function of the inner ear and diseases affecting it continues to be incomplete.

What the future looks like.
- MRI testing techniques capable of looking at the inner ear will aid in making a diagnosis and following the effects of treatment.

- A prosthetic vestibular inner ear that may replace vestibular inner ear function or be used to stop an attack in progress.

- Increased use of drugs like steroids placed directly into the middle ear.

- Basic research will continue to slowly open up more secrets of the inner ear

PREFACE

Ménière's disease was first described in the mid-1800's by the French physician, Prosper Ménière. Although it's been around all this time, confusion and controversy still swirl around it. It continues to be a very frustrating, confusing, frightening, highly stressful addition to the hectic modern life.

This book has been written to quickly put Ménière's information into the hands of those who need it most, people who have it. According to the National Institutes of Health that's 615,000 people in the U.S. with 45,500 new cases added yearly.

"I was author of the 1998 book, "Ménière's Disease: What You Need to Know," but this is not a second edition of that book. There has been no collaboration with the Vestibular Disorders Association or it's medical advisors. Every page, from first to last, has been written independently with up to date information and the central goal of providing a concise, affordable book.

This book can't fix Ménière's but the information about what it is, what it does, how it's diagnosed, and how it's treated as well as ideas for coping may ease the uncertainty, confusion, frustration, and stress, a bit.

If you have Ménière's, use this book as a tool to help understand what your healthcare provider is telling you, to make informed decisions about your care and to live on with the disorder. Please don't use it as a substitute for individualized medical advice and care.

This book is written to give insight into how "main stream" health care deals with Ménière's disease. Every chapter has a reference list at the end containing titles of all the books, scientific journal articles and websites used as sources in preparing this book.

REFERENCES:
http://www.nidcd.nih.gov/health/balance Accessed Oct 3, 2017.

Ménière's Disease Explained

CHAPTER ONE
WHAT IS MÉNIÈRE'S DISEASE?

Since 1995 the American Association of Otolaryngology-Head and Neck Surgery (AAOHNS), the largest organization of doctors treating Ménière's in the U.S., has defined Ménière's as the "idiopathic syndrome of endolymphatic hydrops" and calls it Ménière's disease.

- *Idiopathic*
This means the cause of a disease isn't known. Over the years many ideas about the cause of Ménière's disease have been discussed including adrenal-pituitary insufficiency, allergy, autoimmune disorder, autonomic nervous system malfunction, bacterial infection, channelapathy, cholesterol elevation, circulation disorder, dental issues, ear trauma, endolymph blockage, gluten allergy, ischemia (lack of oxygen to parts of the inner ear), malformed or small endolymphatic sac, head trauma, heredity/genetics, hormonal imbalance, dislodged otoconia (ear rocks), hyperinsulinemia, menstrual or premenstrual problems, mental health issues, migraine, otosclerosis, loud sound/noise trauma, prolactinoma, stress, structural abnormality, thyroid disease, trauma and viral infection but the cause continues to be unknown.

- *Syndrome*
A group of signs and symptoms occurring in a pattern is a syndrome whereas a disease is a physical or chemical change in the way the body or mind functions. This means a syndrome is defined by its symptoms and a disease is defined by the change that has caused it.

Ménière's disease or Ménière's syndrome? Although the AAOHNS calls it Ménière's disease there are other terms in use by various physicians including cochlear Ménière's disease and Ménière's syndrome. Those who use the term syndrome usually do so when the cause is unknown and disease when it is known. When only hearing symptoms are present some physicians use the term cochlear Ménière's. Although in use these terms are not in line with the American Association of Otolaryngology-Head and Neck Surgery (AAOHNS).

- *Endolymphatic hydrops*
This is an increased amount of endolymphatic fluid in the inner ear. Ménière's disease has been linked to endolymphatic hydrops since 1938 when physicians in Britain and Japan first found hydrops in the ears of a few people who had the symptoms of Ménière's disease during their lives.

1

Note: The only way then, and now, to see and actually measure endolymphatic hydrops is to remove the skull bone containing the inner ear, prepare it with chemicals for a period of time and view it with a microscope. It cannot be detected with absolute certainty in a living person but this is changing as MRI techniques better able to see the inner ear transition from research to clinical practice.

Since 1938 endolymphatic hydrops has been considered the result of Ménière's disease and possibly the cause of its symptoms. This physical change in the ear has been the target of many treatments, both medical and surgical.

Now, a newer view of Ménière's is emerging and gaining some support: whatever causes the Ménière's disease also causes the increase in endolymph, that they are two effects from one cause and not cause and effect.

Why the slow change in thought? Basic scientific research has found both endolymphatic hydrops in the ears of people who did not have the symptoms of Ménière's during their lives and no endolymphatic hydrops in some people who did have the symptoms of Ménière's. Another consideration is that treatments to improve Ménière's disease aimed at the reduction of endolymph fail in a significant number of people (1/3 is often quoted in the medical literature). When they do help they usually fail to improve the hearing loss, tinnitus and aural fullness.

In short, Ménière's is a chronic, incurable, nonfatal disorder of the inner ear whose main symptoms are vertigo, hearing loss, ringing in the ears and/or a feeling of ear fullness. But there's a lot more to this disorder than that short description. Although the symptoms were first attributed to the inner ear by the French physician Prosper Ménière back in the 1800's, we still don't know what causes it so its diagnosis and treatment remain difficult. Some doctors even speculate that Ménière's is a name used for a number of different conditions and isn't a single disease.

It can develop in all races and sexes as well as in children, octogenarians, astronauts, street sweepers, rich, poor, the healthy, and the not so healthy, the famous and the ordinary. Studies around the world have found the most common starting age for Ménière's is between 40 and 49 years with slightly more women developing it than men. According to the National Institutes of Health around 615,000 people in the U.S. have a diagnosis of Ménière's with 45,500 new cases added each year. The National Institute for Health and Care Excellence of the UK estimates that 1 in 1000 Britain's have the disorder.

There is some evidence that it occurs more often in people of European ancestry.

The number of people with Ménière's disease differs greatly from one study to another. The table below gives a summary of worldwide studies.

NUMBERS WITH MÉNIÈRE'S	RESEARCHER	COUNTRY	YEAR
157/100,000	Cawthorne, Hewlett	UK	1954
218 / 100,000	Wladislavosky-Waserman	US	1953-1980
46 / 100,000	Stahle	Sweden	1978
205 /100,000	Celestino, Ralli	Italy	1991
21.4-36 / 100,000	Shojaku	Japan	1997
43 / 100,000	Kotimaki	Finland	1999
25/11,463	Ibekwe/Jaduola	Nigeria	2007
120 / 100,000	Radtke	Germany	2008
190 / 100,000	Harris	US	2010

None of these studies is perfect, all have drawbacks. For example, the 2010 study looked at health insurance data, leaving out all people who didn't have insurance. In the older studies people were counted as having Ménière's who would not now meet the strict diagnostic definition. Both the National Institutes of Health (USA) and the National Health System (UK) figures are estimates, not actual head counts.

One British study has estimated Ménière's disease costs the UK £541,000 to £608,700 per year or £3,342 to £3,757 per person, per year.

TREND
These days more people are being diagnosed with Vestibular Migraine, also called Migraine Associated Vertigo, who in the past would have been labeled with Ménière's disease. This is most likely to be the case in a person with a history of headaches, migraine or family history of migraine.

3

SIMILAR DISORDERS

Ménière's disease isn't the only disease of the inner ear. There are many other disorders that can cause some similar symptoms and distress including:

Acoustic neuroma: Non-cancerous tumor of the vestibular branch of the vestibulocochlear nerve that may also involve the hearing and facial nerves. (Keep in mind that tumors are one of the *least* likely causes of Ménière's-like symptoms).

Bacterial labyrinthitis: Bacterial infection of the inner ear usually causing vertigo, hearing loss and possibly tinnitus (ringing in the ears).

Benign paroxysmal vertigo of childhood: A migraine condition of young children with sudden, short attacks of vertigo.

Cholesteatoma: Middle ear mass, usually from chronic middle ear infections, made of cholesterol and epithelium (type of tissue) that can erode away surrounding structures.

Delayed endolymphatic hydrops: Type of endolymphatic hydrops in which symptoms start years apart.

Endolymphatic hydrops: Greater than normal amount of endolymph in the inner ear.

Enlarged vestibular aqueduct syndrome: Structural problem of the inner ear in which the vestibular aqueduct is too large.

Labyrinthitis: General name for any inflammation (redness and swelling) of the inner ear.

Migraine associated vertigo: Vertigo caused by a migraine that may or may not include a headache. An excellent article can be found in the *Neurologic Clinics, 33*(3):619-628, 2015.

Otosclerosis: Abnormal bone growth on the inner ear's bony covering and/or on the little stapes middle ear bone.

Ototoxicity: Inner ear poisoning from drugs or chemicals.

Perilymphatic fistula (PLF): Abnormal opening between the middle and inner ears allowing the escape of perilymph into the middle ear, or an abnormal opening between the perilymph containing area of the inner ear and the endolymph containing area.

Shingles of the ear: Herpes zoster viral infection of the vestibulocochlear nerve.

Superior canal dehiscence: Bone abnormality in which the superior semicircular canal is not totally covered by the temporal bone.

Syphilis of the ear: Syphilis that has spread to the inner ear.

Vascular loop syndrome: Squeezing or compression of the vestibulocochlear nerve by a blood vessel.

Vertebrobasilar insufficiency or occlusion: Decreased blood flow to the brain, inner ear and/or vestibulocochlear nerve.

Vestibular neuronitis: Viral infection/inflammation of the vestibular branch of the vestibulocochlear nerve.

Viral labyrinthitis: Viral infection/inflammation of the inner ear.

Von Hippel-Lindau disease: Genetic disease that can occasionally affect the inner ear in addition to other body areas.

REFERENCES:

Alexander, T.H. and Harris, J.P. "Current epidemiology of Ménière's disease." *Otolaryngological Clinics of North America, 43:*965-970, 2010.

Berlinger, N.T. "Ménière's disease: new concepts, new treatments." *Minnesota Medicine, 94*(11):33-36, 2011.

Brantberg, K., Duan, M. and Falahat, B. "Meniere's disease in children aged 4-7 years." *Acta Oto-Laryngologica, 132:*505-509, 2012.

Brenner, M., Hoistad, D.L. and Hain, T.C. "Prevalence of Thyroid Dysfunction in Patients With Ménière's Disease." *Archives of Otolaryngology-Head and Neck Surgery, 130:*226-228, 2004.

Cawthorne, T. and Hewlett, A.B. "Ménière's disease." *Proceedings of the Royal Society of Medicine, 47:*663-670, 1954.

Celestino, D. and Ralli, G. "Incidence of Ménière's disease in Italy." *American Journal of Otology, 12:*135-138, 1991.

Committee on Hearing and Equilibrium. "Committee on Hearing and Equilibrium Guidelines for the Diagnosis and Evaluation of Therapy in Ménière's Disease." *Otolaryngology-Head and Neck Surgery, 113*(3):181-185, 1995.

D'Avila, C. and Lavinsky, L. "Glucose and insulin profiles and their correlations in Ménière's disease." *International Tinnitus Journal, 11*(2):170-176, 2005.

Derebery, M.J. and Berliner, K.I. "Allergy and Ménière's Disease." *Current Allergy and Asthma Reports, 6:*451-456, 2007.

Di Berardino, F. and Cesarani, A. "Gluten sensitivity in Meniere's disease." *Laryngoscope, 122*(3):700-702, 2012.

Eidelman, D. "Ménière's disease may be caused by common intraosseous dental pathology--Diagnosis using the comparative compression sign." *Medical Hypotheses, 68*(2):389-392, 2007.

Fattori, B., Nacci, A., Darden, A., Dallan, I., Grosso, M., Traino, C., Mancini, V., Ursino, F. and Monzani, F. "Possible association between thyroid autoimmunity and Ménière's disease." *Clinical and Experimental Immunology, 152:*28-32, 2008.

Foster, C.A. and Breeze, R.E. "The Ménière's attack: an ischemia/reperfusion disorder of inner ear sensory tissues." *Medical Hypotheses, 81*(6):1108-1115, 2013.

Gates, P. "Hypothesis: could Ménière's disease be a channelopathy?" *Internal Medicine Journal, 35:*488–489, 2005.

Goebel, J. "2015 Equilibrium Committee Amendment to the 1995 AAO-HNS Guidelines for the Definition of Ménière's Disease." *Otolaryngology-Head and Neck Surgery,* 154(3):403-404, 2016.

Harris, J.P. and Nguyen, Q.T., "Ménière's Disease." *Otolaryngology Clinics of North America, 43*(5):965-1142, 2010.

Hallpike, C. S. and Cairns, H.W. "Observations on the pathology of Ménière's syndrome." *Proceedings of the Royal Society of Medicine, 31:*1317-1336, 1938.

Hinchcliffe, R. "Personality Profile in Ménière's Disease." *Journal of Laryngology and Otology, 81*(5):477-481, 1967.

Hoffer, M., Gottshall, K., Balough, B., Wester, D. and Moore, R. "The Etiology and Pathophysiology of Post-Traumatic Endolymphatic Hydrops." ARO abstract 579 – 2007 mid-winter meeting, accessed January 21, 2013. http://www.aro.org/mwm/07_Abstract_Book.pdf

Horner, K.C., Guieu, R., Magnan, J., Chays, A. and Cazals, Y. "Prolactinoma in some Ménière's Patients —is stress involved? *Neuropsychopharmacology*, *26*:135–138, 2002.

Hornibrook, J. and Bird, P. "A new theory for Meniere's disease." *Otolaryngology-Head and Neck Surgery,*156(2):350-352, 2017.

Ibekwe, T.S. and Ijaduola, G.T. "Ménière's disease: rare or underdiagnosed among Africans*?*" *European Archives of Otorhinolaryngology, 264*(12):1399-1403, 2007.

Kotimaki, J., Sorri, M., Aantaa, E. and Nuutinen, J. "Prevalence of Ménière's disease in Finland." *Laryngoscope, 109*(5):748-753, 1999.

Merchant, S.N., Adams, J.C. and Nadol, J.B. "Pathophysiology of Ménière's syndrome: are symptoms caused by endolymphatic hydrops?" *Otology and Neurotology, 26(*1):74-81, 2005.

Nakagawa, H., Ohashi, N., Kanda, K. and Watanabe, Y. "Autonomic Nervous System Disturbance as Etiological Background of Vertigo and Dizziness." *Acta Otolaryngologica, Supplement, 504*:130-133, 1993.

Nakashima, T., Naganawa, S., Sugiura, M., Teranishi, M., Sone, M., Hayashi, H., Nakata, S., Katayama, N. and Ishida, I.M. "Visualization of endolymphatic hydrops in patients with Ménière's disease." *Laryngoscope, 117*(3):415-420, 2007.

NICE, Clinical Knowledge Summary, http://cks.nice.org.uk/menieres-disease#!topicsummary, Accessed May, 2017.

NIDCD http://www.nidcd.nih.gov/health/balance Accessed June, 2017.

Ohmen, J.D., White, C.H., Li, X., Wang, J., Fisher, L.M., Zhang, H., Derebery, M.J. and Friedman, R.A. "Genetic evidence for an ethnic diversity in the susceptibility to Ménière's disease." *Otology and Neurotology, 34*(7):1336-1341, 2013.

Pappas, D.G. and Banyas, J.B. "A Newly Recognized Etiology of Ménière's Syndrome: A Preliminary Report." *Acta Otolaryngologica, Supplement, 485*:104-107, 1991.

Parker, W. "Ménière's Disease: Etiologic Considerations." *Archives of Otolaryngology-Head and Neck Surgery, 121*:377-382, 1995.

Radtke, A., von Brevern, M., Feldmann, M., Lezius, F., Zeise, T., Lempert, T. and Neuhauser, H. "Screening for Ménière's disease in the general population - the needle in the haystack." *Acta Otolaryngologica, 128*:272-276, 2008.

Rauch, S.D., Merchant, S.N. and Thedinger, B.A. "Ménière's syndrome and endolymphatic hydrops. Double-blind temporal bone study." *Annals of Otology Rhinology and Laryngology, 98*(11):873-883, 1989.

Rauch, S.D. "Clinical Hints and Precipitating Factors in Patients Suffering from Ménière's Disease." *Otolaryngological Clinics of North America, 43*(5):1011-1017, 2010.

Seemungal, B., Kaski, D. and Lopez-Escamez, J.A. "Early diagnosis and management of acute vertigo from vestibular migraine and Ménière's disease." *Neurologic Clinics, 33*(3):619-628, 2015.

Shojaku, H. and Watanabe, Y. "The prevalence of definite cases of Ménière's disease in the Hida and Nishikubiki districts of central Japan: a survey of relatively isolated areas of medical care." *Acta Otolaryngologica Supplement, 528*:94-96, 1997.

Stahle, J., Stahle, C. and Arenberg, I. K. "Incidence of Ménière's disease." *Archives of Otolaryngology, 104*(2):99-102, 1978.

Tyrrell, J., Whinney, D.J. And Taylor, T. "The cost of Meniere's Disease: a novel multisource approach." *Ear and Hearing, 35*(4):162-169, 2014.

Wladislavosky-Waserman, P., Facer, G.W., Mokri, B. and Kurland, L.T. "Ménière's Disease: a 30-Year Epidemiologic and Clinical Study in Rochester, Minn., 1951-1980." *Laryngoscope, 94*:1098-1102, 1984.

Yamakawa, K. "Uber die pathologische Veranderung bei einem Meniere-Kranken." *Journal of Otolaryngology Japan, 44*:2310-2312, 1938.

Yazawa, Y., Suzuki, M., Hanamitsu, M., Kimura, H. and Tooyama, I. "Detection of viral DNA in the endolymphatic sac in Ménière's disease by in situ hybridization." *Journal of Otorhinolaryngology and Related Specialties, 65*(3):162-168, 2003.

CHAPTER TWO
THE EAR AND HOW IT WORKS

To understand the changes associated with Ménière's disease, and how treatments are thought to work, its useful to know something about the ear's structure and function as well as how the brain both uses information from the inner ear and carries out balance.

Our ears are divided into three areas, the external ear, middle ear and inner ear and have two functions, hearing and vestibular function (balance function). All three ear areas participate in hearing, only the inner ear has a role in both hearing and vestibular function. The inner ear is also the only area affected by Ménière's disease.

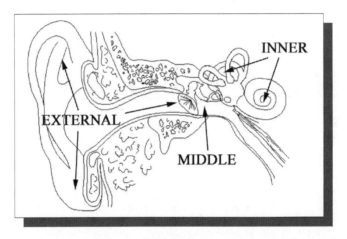

Vestibular function is not all there is to balance and balance needs more than vestibular function. Vestibular information is needed for efficient balance to take place as well as some other functions.

While reading about the inner ear's structure and function keep in mind that a great deal remains undiscovered since it's difficult and expensive to study. As new discoveries are made and our understanding of the ear increases, the information written here will change, perhaps even dramatically.

STRUCTURE
• External ear: Has two parts, the outside flap (auricle) and the ear canal

(external auditory canal).

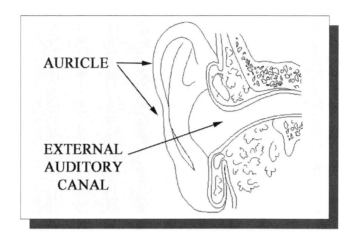

- Middle ear: Has several parts, the ear drum (tympanic membrane), middle ear cavity, three little ear bones (ossicles), eustachian tube, and two membrane covered openings between it and the inner ear. It's three little bones (malleus, incus and stapes) form a chain through the middle ear cavity from the ear drum to the membrane-covered hole into the inner ear called the oval window. The eustachian tube connects the middle ear to the throat area behind the nose.

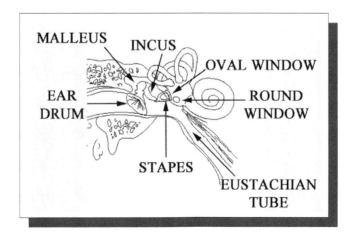

- Inner ear: This pea-sized organ is located inside the temporal bone, a solid bone that's part of the skull. It has three areas, the cochlea, vestibule and semicircular canals. There are two more balance structures inside the vestibule, the utricle and saccule. The saccule is very close to the oval window, the membrane covered opening between the middle and inner ear. The close proximity of the saccule to the stapes bone can be a factor in the creation of symptoms.

Two chemically different fluids, perilymph and endolymph, fill the inner ear. The areas holding this fluid are located one inside the other and separated by a membrane with endolymph in the middle and perilymph surrounding it.

The endolymphatic duct, endolymphatic sac and the vestibulo-cochlear nerve are all connected to the inner ear. The endolymphatic duct connects the inner ear with the endolymphatic sac. Unlike the rest of the inner ear, the sac is not totally encased by the temporal bone and is located very close to the brain. The sac is also the target of endolymphatic sac surgery.

One nerve, the vestibulo-cochlear nerve, also called the acoustic nerve and the 8th cranial nerve, connects the inner ear directly to the brain. It has two parts or branches, the vestibular and the cochlear. This nerve passes through a tunnel in the temporal bone before entering an area around the brain. It shares this tunnel with another nerve, the facial nerve. The fact that the vestibulo-cochlear nerve and facial nerve travel together becomes important if surgery to cut the nerve is ever considered.

FUNCTION
All structures in the ear perform specific tasks. Some parts are directly involved in hearing or vestibular function while others have a more supportive role to play in keeping the ear functioning. The external and middle ears are only involved in hearing while the inner ear is involved in both hearing and balance.

Vestibular function
Information about both our position in space and movement are collected by the five vestibular structures; saccule, utricle and three semicircular canals. The three semicircular canals sense circular movement that's increasing or decreasing in speed and the utricle and saccule sense movement in a straight line that is increasing or decreasing in speed as well as sensing gravity. Movement or position change bends specific hair cells in the inner ear.

This creates a chemical reaction sending signals to the brain via the vestibulo-cochlear nerve. The brain evaluates which hair cells have been bent and determines position in space along with movement from this information. It can do this in part because the vestibular structures are embedded in the temporal bone so their location within the ear does not change.

In addition to balance, vestibular information is used to keep vision clear during head movement, maintain blood pressure when first standing and respiratory muscle adjustments during changes in position. All these functions are carried out rapidly and without our conscious involvement via reflexes.

The vestibular reflexes are the vestibulo-ocular reflex (VOR), vestibulo-spinal reflex (VSR), vestibulo-cervical reflex (VCR) and the vestibulo-autonomic reflexes.

A reflex is an automatic neurological connection between a stimulus and the reaction to it. The same stimulus always brings on the same reaction. A familiar reflex is the knee jerk, when the lower leg kicks forward after the tendon on the front of the knee is tapped with a little hammer. Tapping is the stimulus and lower leg movement is the reaction. Tapping the right knee always brings on movement of the right lower leg, each time, every time, unless the reflex is damaged.

Standing balance is the task of the VSR. The brain receives vestibular information, sends commands to the appropriate muscles of the neck, trunk, arms, and legs, making them contract and relax in the proper sequence to keep us upright.

The task of both the VOR and VCR is to prevent the jumping or blurring of vision during head movement. The VOR does this by moving the eyes in response to head movement. When vision is absent (in darkness or with the eyes closed), turning the head in one direction results in movement of the eyes at exactly the same time and rate of speed in the opposite direction. The VCR sends commands to neck muscles that keep the head in the proper position for the eyes to remain fixed on a target of interest. It also helps keep the head in a vertical position, i.e. stops you from tilting your head at the wrong time.

The vestibulo-autonomic (or vestibulo-sympathetic) reflexes use information about position and movement to help maintain blood pressure in the milliseconds after we stand up and to adjust respiratory muscles as we move around. The respiratory rate can be increased, the depth of each breath can be deepened, and both the diaphragm and chest muscles can be changed through this reflex.

Balance

Balance is a complicated function requiring information from a number of sources as well as the work of many body parts. There must be an alert mind, intact spinalcord, strong muscles and flexible joints for balance to be successful. In addition, practice and experience in all our physical activities are needed as well as knowing what to expect. Information comes from the vestibular areas of the inner ear, vision and proprioception.

- The inner ear supplies information about our movement, position in space and the effect of gravity.

- Proprioception is a system of pressure sensors scattered around the skeletal muscles, tendons, joints, ligaments, and the connective tissue covering the bones and muscles. These sensors collect information about gravity, position, surfaces, and stretch and motion of the muscles and joints. This information is used to determine what movement is being undertaken and where different body parts are in relationship to one another. Proprioception is needed to find the tip of your nose with your finger when your eyes are closed, for example. It's also used to feel the ground when standing.

- Vision helps with balance by filling in some gaps in vestibular information. Vision supplies information about our movement at a steady speed, something the inner ear can't sense. Movement can be sensed by seeing objects grow larger while moving toward them and smaller when moving away. Vision gives us information about the location of horizontal and vertical and can help determine if the head is moving alone or if the body and head are moving together.

All three senses are needed for the best balance function because each provides some basic information that the others don't. Because there is a great deal of overlapping information collected, balance can take place with information from only two. An example of this is in total darkness, when vision isn't available, someone with normal proprioception and vestibular function can usually remain upright and move about without falling.

Hearing

The ear collects sound waves, turns them into electric signals and sends the signals to the brain. Sound waves enter the ear in one of two ways, traveling through the skull to the middle ear or being collected and funneled through the external ear to the middle ear. When funneled in through the external ear the sound waves move the eardrum in and out. This movement is carried through the middle ear cavity along the little ear bones, the ossicles. The first ossicle is connected to the eardrum and the third bone, the stapes, is connected to the oval window, a membrane covered opening into the inner ear. Movement of the eardrum causes all three bones to move and the stapes to push the oval window in and out.

Movement into the ear:

Eardrum → Malleus → Incus → Stapes → Oval Window

Oval window movement produces a movement of fluid in the cochlea called the traveling wave. As the wave travels through the cochlea, hair cells are bent. This bending causes a chemical reaction sending signals through the vestibulo-cochlear nerve to the brain where they can be recognized as sound and acted upon if necessary.

Movement out of the ear:

Oval Window → Stapes →   Incus → Malleus → Eardrum

Supporting roles

Eustachian tube

The middle ear cavity must be kept at the same pressure as the external ear for the eardrum to move freely. Maintaining the proper pressure is the job of the eustachian tube that runs from the throat to the middle ear. Every time we yawn or swallow the tube opens letting outside air into the middle ear so pressure can equalize.

A cold or sinus infection can prevent the eustachian tube from opening and the pressure from equalizing. Failure to equalize can cause pain in the short term and both fluid in the middle ear cavity and damage to the middle ear structures over the long term. Some people with Ménière's disease also experience an increase in symptoms when unable to equalize pressure. There are some studies out of Europe implicating poor eustachian tube function as a symptom causer in Ménière's disease.

Endolymphatic Sac

Traditionally the sac was thought of as the place endolymph flowed to at the end of its trip through the inner ear. It's now known that endolymph doesn't normally flow through the inner ear this way, it's made and disposed of in many locations throughout it. The sac is probably both an immune and lymph organ carrying out functions like the production and reabsorption of endolymph locally, fighting foreign substances, disposing of waste products and may synthesize, secrete, absorb and digest proteins. When the normal fluid state of the inner ear is disturbed the sac may also work to return the fluids to normal. The sac is the target of one surgery for Ménière's disease, endolymphatic sac decompression.

Dark cells

These cells are dark because they contain the pigment melanin. They are located in the vestibular areas and produce endolymph, concentrate and transport potassium and regulate calcium. Proper chemical balance of electrolytes, like potassium, is crucial for both hearing and vestibular function to take place.

Stria vascularis

The cochlear structure producing endolymph as well as concentrating and transporting potassium into the endolymph.

THE DAMAGE OF MÉNIÈRE'S DISEASE

When the ear with endolymphatic hydrops is studied after death, ripped membranes, hair cell disintegration, and structures ripped from their foundations are seen throughout the inner ear. This damage is the reason for the hearing loss, hearing distortions, temporary and/or permanent problems with equilibrium, eye movement, neck movement, and body movement.

REFERENCES:

Baloh, R. and Honrubia,V. *Clinical Neurophysiology of the Vestibular System,* 4th edition. New York: Oxford University Press, 2010.

Gloddek, B. and Arnold, W. "The endolymphatic sac receives antigenetic information from the organs of the musoca-associated lymphatic system." *Acta Otolaryngologica, 118*(3):333-336, 1998.

Guyton, A.C. and Hall, J.E. *Guyton and Hall Textbook of Medical Physiology.* 11th edition. Philadelphia: W.B. Saunders, 2010.

Hallpike, C.S. and Cairns, H. "Observations on the pathology of Meniere's syndrome," *Journal of Laryngology and Otology, 53:*625-655, 1938.

Hebbar, G.K., Rask-Andersen, H. and Linthicum, F.H. "Three-dimensional analysis of 61 human endolymphatic ducts and sacs in ears with and without Ménière's disease." *Annals of Otology-Rhinology and Laryngology, 100*(3):219-225, 1991.

Hitier, M., Besnard, S. and Smith, P.F. "Vestibular pathways involved in cognition." *Frontiers in Integrated Neuroscience, 23*;8:59. doi: 10.3389/fnint.2014.00059. eCollection 2014.

Khan, S. and Chang, R. "Anatomy of the vestibular system: a review." *NeuroRehabilitation, 32(3*):437-443, 2013.

Leigh, R.J. and Zee, D.S. *The Neurology of Eye Movements* 4th edition, New York:Oxford University Press, 2006.

Marieb, E.N. and Hoehn, K. *Human Anatomy and Physiology 9th edition.* London:Pearson, 2012.

Ovortrup, K., Rostgaard, J., Holstein-Rathlou, N.H. and Bretlau, P. "The endolymphatic sac, a potential endocrine gland?" *Acta Otolaryngologica, 119*(2):194-199, 1999.

Salt, A.N. "Regulation of endolymphatic fluid volume." *Annals of the New York Academy of Science, 942:*306-312, 2001.

Tascioglu, A.B. "Brief review of vestibular system anatomy and its higher order projections." *Neuroanatomy, 4:*24-27, 2005.

Weber, P.C. *Vertigo and disequilibrium: A practical guide to diagnosis and management.* Thieme:New York, 2005.

Yates, B.J. and Bronstein, A.M. "The effects of vestibular system lesions on autonomic regulation: Observations, mechanisms, and clinical implications." *Journal of Vestibular Research, 15:*119-129, 2005.

CHAPTER THREE
SIGNS AND SYMPTOMS

Ménière's disease can produce a staggering array of symptoms falling into two broad categories, the major or diagnostic symptoms and all the others.

MAJOR SYMPTOMS
The major symptoms have always defined Ménière's disease. Their presence is the only diagnostic criteria suggested by the Committee on Balance and Equilibrium of the American Academy of Otolaryngology-Head and Neck Surgery (AAOHNS). These diagnostic symptoms are episodic vertigo, hearing loss, ear fullness and ringing in the ears.

- *Vertigo* is the perception of movement that is not occurring or is occurring differently from what is perceived. The vertigo of Ménière's disease can be violent and last 20 minutes to 24 hours with episodes occurring again and again in frustratingly unpredictable intervals. It's also spontaneous, coming out of the blue, not because a person shook their head, looked up at the top shelf, watched a moving object or any other activity. Vertigo, and the uncertainty it brings, is also the symptom having the biggest impact on quality of life.

- *Hearing loss* may be constant, fluctuate or occur only with the vertigo episodes. More hearing may be lost with each attack of vertigo. This hearing loss is nerve loss, also called sensorineural hearing loss, meaning the damage is in the inner ear, not in the middle ear. Low-pitched sounds are usually affected first with high-pitched sounds being lost later in the disease. Hearing loss usually does not progress to complete deafness but can affect the ability to hear and understand the spoken word.

- *Ear fullness* or pressure, also called aural fullness, is experienced by 25 to 75% of people with Ménière's disease. Just like hearing loss it can be constant, fluctuate or occur only with the vertigo. It may also worsen with each episode of vertigo. This appears as one of the first symptoms in 45% of people, considered the worst symptom in 4.4%, severe for 38% and worse for women, in one study.

- *Ringing in the ears*, also called tinnitus, can be constant, fluctuate or occur only with the vertigo. It may worsen during episodes of vertigo.

The sound is usually low pitched and described as a roaring, blowing, buzzing, crickets chirping or radio static sound. It may be more or less constant in the later years of the disorder.

OTHER SYMPTOMS
There are a large number of other symptoms possible in Ménière's disease. None of these symptoms are specific to it, they can and do occur in other diseases as well. Symptoms can be found below:

General		
Drunk feeling	Insecurity	Neckache
Fatigue	Loss feeling	Sea sickness
Frustration	Malaise	Sleepiness
Hangover feeling	Motion sickness	Spaced out feeling
Balance		
Clumsiness	Motion sickness	Touching things while walking
Grabbing for stable objects when walking	Motion intolerance	Trouble turning
Looking down while walking	Staggering Stumbling	Unsteadiness
Thought and memory		
Easily distracted	Loss of self-esteem	Slurred speech
Groping for words	Loss of self-Reliance	Trouble concentrating
Loss of self-confidence	Short-term memory difficulties	Worry
Feelings		
Anger/rage	Failure	Self-blame
Depression, Sadness	Guilt	Shame
Embarrassment	Loss of control	
Fear, anxiety		
Anxiety	Fear	Rapid pulse
Cold sweat	Hyperventilation	Perspiration
Diarrhea	Palpitations	Tension
		Trembling
Head		
Headache	Heavy headedness	Lightheadedness (faintness)

Gastrointestinal		
Malaise	Poor appetite	Stiffneck
Nausea	Queasiness	Stiffness
	Sleep disturbance	Vomiting
Sound		
Sound distortion	Sound sensitivity	Tullio phenomenon
Vision		
Blurred vision	Eye jerking	Trouble reading
Bouncing vision	Intensified glare	Trouble watching movement
Difficulty focusing	Jerking of vision	Visual distortions
Difficulty in visually busy areas	Poor depth Perception	

HOW ARE THE OTHER SYMPTOMS PRODUCED?

Symptoms are caused by a number of things, including temporary chemical changes inside the ear, disruption of the vestibular reflexes, permanent damage from chemical changes or excess endolymph fluid, change in self-perception and a change in the way people are viewed by others.

- *Anger* can come from feeling so horrible, the loss of function and the interruption to life.

- *Cold sweat and anxiety* come from the autonomic nervous system, the nervous system regulating the body's automatic functions. It revs up during an attack producing anxiety, blurred vision, cold sweat, dry mouth, goose bumps, hyperventilation, racing heart, and trembling because it views a Ménière's attack as an emergency. The uncertainty of Ménière's disease leads to anxiety as does the interference with vestibular reflexes.

- *Depression* comes from having an unpredictable, chronic, potentially disabling illness. It can also appear due to physical changes such as dehydration.

- *Ear fullness* might be caused by the excess endolymph fluid in the inner ear.

- *Ear ringing,* or tinnitus, probably comes from both cochlear damage and the resulting hearing loss but the exact change or changes for this and other causes of ear ringing are unknown.

- *Fatigue and malaise* come from the energy used during the attack, particularly from the autonomic nervous system response and from vomiting/retching. In the days after the attack, maintaining balance requires more effort while the brain reorganizes and becomes accustomed to any permanent change and possibly begins to rely more upon vision and proprioception for balance. A hearing loss, causes a tiring struggle to hear things as well.

- *Fear and worry* about when and where the next attack will occur, if falling and/or injury will occur, how people will view them, and embarrassment; fear and worry about money making and bill paying abilities. Long-term stress can cause this as well.

- *Headaches* can be caused by just plain not feeling well, facial muscle strain from trying to focus the eyes, holding the head rigidly during an attack, and vomiting.

- *Lightheadedness and heavyheadedness* can be caused by irritation or damage to the inner ear's gravity sensing areas. Lightheadedness can also result from dehydration and the autonomic nervous system response.

- *Memory, concentration and other thought problems* probably result from the amount of attention balance now requires and the interference with the vestibular reflexes.

- *Motion sickness* can occur anytime information from vision, proprioception and the vestibular areas of the inner ears don't match.

- *Muscle stiffness* from holding the neck rigidly to prevent head movement during an attack, vomiting and dry heaves, laying in bed for hours and the disruption to the vestibular reflexes controlling movement and the neck muscles.

- *Nausea and vomiting* are common during an attack because vestibular information is shared with the brain's vomiting center.

- *Poor appetite* comes from not feeling well, the nausea and vomiting during the attack, lingering nausea and/or a digestive system slowdown caused by the autonomic nervous system. It can also come from long-term stress.

- *Sound distortion and sensitivity* come from problems in the cochlea, perhaps from the excess endolymph.

- *Tullio phenomenon* is vertigo occurring during sound, usually loud sound. This may come from the middle ear's stapes bone pushing on the oval window into a very swollen and sensitive saccule.

- *Tumarkin's otolithic crisis* is a sudden fall due to complete loss of balance, without vertigo. It's thought to be produced by a sudden, complete loss of the saccule's gravity sensing ability more common in later Ménière's disease. More later in this chapter.

"In MD, there seem to exist a vicious circle of interaction between the somatic symptoms especially vertigo and resultant emotional disturbances, which in turn tend to provoke some other somatic symptoms. The quality of life of the sufferers is severely incapacitated by the illness, especially the psychological well-being, which manifest mainly with anxiety and depression, dominating the physical and environmental disturbances. Worse quality of life tends to occur in Ménière's patients with more severe vertigo symptom."

EARLY MÉNIÈRE'S DISEASE
In the beginning the Ménière's disease experience is usually a repeating sequence of symptoms appearing at unpredictable time intervals. The sequence of events may include the warning, attack, aftermath and remission.

Warning
As many as 50 percent of people with Ménière's disease experience symptoms or sensations immediately before an attack. It's unknown if the warning is the beginning of an inner ear change that worsens into an attack or if it's one change in the inner ear followed by another change producing more symptoms.

A warning varies from person to person but will usually include one or more of stomach discomfort, heartburn, perspiration, headache, hearing hearing loss or increased hearing loss, ear ringing or increased ear ringing or a change in the character of the ear ringing, ear fullness/pressure or increased pressure, headache, lightheadedness, dizziness, slight balance disturbance, increased sensitivity to sound, and/or a vague feeling of uneasiness -- alone or in any combination. Some people simply feel an attack coming on and cannot really describe what they are feeling.

Visual symptoms like flashing lights or sudden blindness are not part of a Ménière's warning nor are fainting, smells, or muscle weakness.

This warning time period is one reason most people with Ménière's disease don't experience serious injuries during an attack. They have time to stop their car, get off the lawnmower, turn off the oven, put down the chainsaw and seek safety before prostrating symptoms strike. There is probably not enough time to land an airplane, bring a boat back to shore or come back from a long hike in the wilderness.

Attack
The "attack" refers to an episode of vertigo that can be accompanied by ear ringing, hearing loss, and ear fullness along with nausea, vomiting, abnormal eye movement, visual disturbances, sweating, rapid heart beat, palpitations, cold sweat, fear, anxiety, trembling, anger, hyperventilation, blurred vision, and more. The vertigo is usually spinning and can be violent, forcing around 83% of people to lay down with only 17% able to carry on with activities during an attack.

Of course during a severe attack balance ability is almost gone. But some people have less severe attacks in which balance is only impaired. During a mild attack of vertigo there will be spatial disorientation, trouble in determining position in three-dimensional space, making walking around difficult and risky.

One attack description from the British Medical Journal: "An attack usually starts with cochlear symptoms followed soon after by the onset of vertigo. The vertigo peaks rapidly in intensity, when patients might be forced to lie still, and diminishes over a period of 20 minutes but not more than 24 hours."

How often does this occur? One study of 243 people found 13% had attacks once or twice a year, 23% had 3-12 attacks each year and 63% had one or more each month with 5% feeling their attacks were nearly continuous.

A great many events, situations, and circumstances have been implicated in setting attacks into motion. Most involve pressure changes, fluid changes and impairment of the inner ear's circulation. Airplane travel, alcohol, caffeine, chocolate, cholesterol increase, cigarettes, fatigue, insomnia, premenstrual fluid retention, salt, stress, sugar, elevated triglycerides, and weather changes are all suspects but they don't cause Ménière's Disease. Instead, Ménière's Disease has caused some change(s) in the inner ear that allows these events and circumstances to become a problem.

A 2017 study of 397 people in the United Kingdom has shown that both symptom severity and attacks increase when humidity is 90% or more and when atmospheric pressure is increased.

Experts feel the attacks of Ménière's disease are caused by some physical or chemical change in the inner ear. Some of their theories include:

- Excess endolymph causing pressure in the ear creating temporary changes that bring on the symptoms. When the amount of endolymph decreases, the pressure decreases and the symptoms stop.

- Ruptures within the inner ear caused by increased endolymph allowing the two inner ear fluids, endolymph and perilymph, to mix irritating nerve endings causing symptoms until the rupture seals shut.

- Intermittent secretion of the endolymphatic sac chemical responsible for drawing excess endolymph into the sac causes an occasional backflow of endolymph into the semicircular canals and cochlea stimulating the hair cells and producing symptoms.

- Asphyxia (no oxygen arriving) possibly caused by the increased fluid pressure.

- Increase in the production of endolymph due to increased amounts of the chemical pADH.

Aftermath

After an attack stops, all symptoms may go away and life can return to normal for some people. In others the ear fullness, hearing loss and ear ringing, continue after the vertigo stops and new symptoms may even appear. These new symptoms range from being a bit tired and drained to

23

disturbances severe enough to stop normal activities for days.

Remission

The remission occurs between the end of the aftermath and the next attack. Otolaryngology textbooks describe this time between attacks of Ménière's disease as free of symptoms or "normal." Unfortunately, this is not always the case. The typical person with Ménière's disease has at least one of the major symptoms, particularly ringing in the ears, all the time and probably has one or more of the others as well.

LATE MÉNIÈRE'S DISEASE

As the disease progresses, the pattern of symptoms changes.Traditionally doctors have spoken of burnout, when the ear is permanently damaged and symptoms stop fluctuating with hearing loss and ringing in the ears becoming permanent, aural fullness lessening and attacks of violent vertigo replaced with a less violent but constant imbalance, unsteadiness and perception of false movement. In the words of Jonathon Swift, author of "Gulliver's Travels," "the giddiness I was subject to, instead of coming seldom and violent, now constantly attends me, more or less, though in a more peaceable manner, yet it will not qualify me to live among the young and the healthy."

Unfortunately this is not always the case. One Finnish study found 36% of people with Ménière's disease for 20 years continued to have 1 to 4 severe attacks weekly. The concept of burnout is based upon the experience and casual observations of individual doctors and a few small studies. There has never been a large-scale, long-term study looking at this issue so the real situation is unknown.

REFERENCES:

Angulo, C.M. and Gallo-Teran, J. "Vestibular drop attacks or Tumarkin's otolithic crisis in patients with Ménière's disease." *Acta Otorhinolarinologica Espanola, 56*(10):469-471, 2005.

Andrews, J.C., Gregory, A.A. and Honrubia, V. "The Exacerbation of Symptoms in Ménière's Disease During the Premenstrual Period." *Archives of Otolaryngology-Head and Neck Surgery, 118*:74-78, 1992.

Baloh, R.W., Jacobson, K. and Winder, T. "Drop attacks with Ménière's syndrome." *Annals of Neurology, 28*(3):384-387, 1990.

Chalat, N.I. "Who was Prosper Meniere and why am I still so dizzy?" *American Journal of Otology, 1*(1):52-56, 1979.

Committee on Hearing and Equilibrium. "Committee on Hearing and Equilibrium Guidelines for the Diagnosis and Evaluation of Therapy in Ménière's Disease." *Otolaryngology-Head and Neck Surgery, 113*(3):181-185, 1995.

Erlandsson, S.I., Eriksson-Mangold, M. and Wiberg, A. "Ménière's disease: Trauma, distress and adaptation studied through focus interview analyses." *Scandinavian Audiology, 25*(Supp 43):45-55, 1996.

Foster, C.A. and Breeze, R.E. "The Meniere attack: an ischemia/reperfusion disorder of inner ear sensory tissues." *Medical Hypotheses, 81*(6):1108-1115, 2013.

Gibson, W.P. and Arenberg, I.K. "The Circulation of Endolymph and a New Theory of the Attacks Occurring in Ménière's Disease." *Surgery of the Inner Ear.* New York: Kugler Publications, 1990.

Gürkov, R., Strobl, R., Heinlin, N., Krause, E., Olzowy, B., and Koppe, C., "Atmospheric Pressure and Onset of Episodes of Meniere's Disease - A Repeated Measures Study." *PLoS ONE* 11(4): e0152714. https://doi.org/10.1371/journal.pone.0152714, 2016.

Halmagyi, G.M., Curthoys, I.S., Colebatch, J.G. and Aw, S.T. "Vestibular responses to sound." *Annals of the New York Academy of Science, 1039*:54-67, 2005.

Harcourt, J., Barrclough, K. and Bronstein, A.M. "Meniere's Disease." *British Medical Journal*, 349: 1756-1833, 2014.

Havia, M. and Kentala, E. "Progression of Symptoms of Dizziness in Ménière's Disease." *Archives of Otolaryngology-Head and Neck Surgery, 130*:431-435, 2004.

Levo, H., Kentala, E., Rasku, J. and Pyykkö, I. "Aural fullness in Ménière's disease." *Audiology and Neurootology, 19*(6):395-399, 2014.

Merchant, S.N., Rauch, S.D. and Nadol, J.B. "Ménière's Disease." *European Archives of Otorhinolaryngology, 252*:63-75, 1995.

Nakayama, M., Suzuki, M., Inagaki, A., Takemura, K., Watanabe, N., Tanigawa, T., Okamoto, K., Hattori, H., Brodie, H. and Murakami, S. "Impaired quality of sleep in Ménière's disease patients." *Journal of Clinical Sleep Medicine, 6*(5):445-449, 2010.

Orji, F. "The Influence of Psychological Factors in Ménière's Disease." *Annals of Medical and Health Sciences Research, 4*(1):3-7, 2014.

Rauch, S. "Clinical Hints and Precipitating Factors in Patients Suffering From Meniere's Disease." *Otolaryngology Clinics of North America, 43*(5):1011-1017, 2010.

Schmidt, W., Sarran, C., Ronan, N., Barrett, G., Whinney, D.J., Fleming, L.E., Osborne, N.J. and Tyrrell, J. "The weather and Meniere's Disease: A longitudinal analysis in the UK." *Otology amd Neurotology:38(2):225-233, 2017.*

Smith, P.F. and Darlington, C.L. "Personality changes in patients with vestibular dysfunction." *Frontiers in Human Neuroscience, 7*(678):1-7, 2013.

Takedo,T., Kakigi, A. and Saito, H. "Antidiuretic Hormone (ADH) and Endolymphatic Hydrops." *Acta Otolaryngologica, Supplement, 519*: 219-222, 1995.

Watson, S.R., Halmagyi, G.M. and Colebatch, J.G. "Vestibular hypersensitivity to sound (Tullio phenomenon): structural and functional assessment." *Neurology, 54*(3):722-728, 2000.

MORE ON TUMARKINS

Another problem can occur in Ménière's disease called Tumarkin's otolithic crisis. This is a sudden, spontaneous drop to the ground, without vertigo, without loss of consciousness or any neurological symptoms, occurring on it's own, not as part of a Ménière's attack. It was first described in the scientific literature in 1936 and is thought to affect somewhere between 6 and 32% of people with Ménière's and may be more common in the elderly.

In one small study, of 40 people, researchers found it occurred for anywhere from one to 14 years, with people experiencing from 1 to 14 episodes. Those experiencing more than one episode usually had them within a one-year period.

The leading theory has been a sudden, total loss of otolothic function. Recent studies with the vestibular evoked myogenic potential test (VEMP) support this theory and further pinpoint the saccule as the affected area. (Otolithic is a term referring to the saccule and utricle, the vestibular organs responsible for sensing increasing and decreasing movement in a straight line as well as gravity.) Normally gravity information from the otoliths is used to initiate muscle action that keeps us upright. Sudden loss of this information stops the muscle commands we depend upon and a fall occurs.

There's absolutely no warning and usually no realization it is occurring because no action is taken to avoid injury. Hitting the floor/ground is usually the first indication there's a problem. If any sensation occurs during this crisis it's typically the feeling of having been pushed to the ground. Because there's no warning, reaching out to avoid or break the fall, rolling, or holding the head up don't occur. If not knocked unconscious or seriously injured people can get up and move about after this because there is no attack of vertigo. There may be a great deal of fear, even trembling, due to the sudden, surprising nature of the event, not unlike a car crash or other traumatic event.

A study from Spain found a higher level of disability and more autonomic nervous system symptoms in people experiencing this problem than those who didn't.

DROP ATTACK
The term "Drop attack" is not a specific diagnosis and has no generally

accepted definition. It seems to be used to describe any body change causing someone to suddenly drop to the ground. It can be brought on by anything causing a loss of consciousness like seizures and brain attacks (stroke), as well as by other conditions that don't cause a loss of consciousness such as the cardiovascular condition hypostatic blood pressure, and, on occasion, by Ménière's disease.

FALLING
Falling isn't typically part of an Ménière's attack because of the warning period. Some unfortunate people get no warning and fall to the ground as their attack begins. During these falls they generally know they are falling and can automatically reach out with their arms to grab hold of something to break their fall or make some defensive movement like rolling or holding their head up to protect themselves. They may not be able to get up or move around until the attack stops.

TESTING
Current research is beginning to show VEMP testing may be useful in determining severity and tracking this problem.

TREATMENT
There is no specific medical treatment for Tumarkin's or drop attacks associated with Ménière's. Destructive surgery such as a nerve section or labyrinthectomy had been recommended in the past but a 2014 study suggests gentamicin injections can be helpful. Researchers found 83.3% of their 24 patients were cured after one injection of the antibiotic gentamicin.

COPING
Hitting the ground is at best unpleasant and at worst dangerous. Life with Tumarkin's is difficult due to the uncertainty of when the next episode might occur and if serious injury will occur. Methods to avoid injury should be discussed completely with a physician. Someone having these events without warning should not drive, pilot an airplane, skipper a boat, go up ladders, work on the roof or any other activity that could cause serious injury during a complete loss of balance.

REFERENCES:

Ballester, M., Liard, P., Vibert, D. and Hausler, R. "Meniere's disease in the elderly." *Otology and Neurotology, 23*(1):73-78, 2002.

Baloh, R.W., Jacobson, K. and Winder, T. "Drop attacks with Meniere's syndrome." *Annals of Neurology, 28*(3):384-387, 1990.

Dallan, I., Bruschini, L., Nacci, A., Bignami, M. and Casani, A.P. "Drop attacks and vertical vertigo after transtympanic gentamicin: diagnosis and management." *Acta Otorhinolaryngologica Italia, 25*(6):370-373, 2005.

Furman, J.M., Cass, S.P. and Whitney, S.L. *Vestibular Disorders: A case-study approach to diagnosis and treatment,* 3rd ed., New York: Oxford University Press, 2008.

Morales, A.C. and Gallo-Teran, J. "Vestibular drop attacks or Tumarkin's otolithic crisis in patients with Meniere's disease." *Acta Otorrinolaringol Espana, 56*(10):469-471, 2005.

Ozeki, H., Iwasaki, S. and Murofushi, T. "Vestibular drop attack secondary to Meniere's disease results from unstable otolithic function." *Acta Oolaryngologica, 128*(8):887-891, 2008.

Perez-Fernandez, N., Montes-Jovellar, L., Cervera-Paz, J. and Domenech-Vadillo, E. "Auditory and vestibular assessment of patients with Ménière's disease who suffer Tumarkin attacks." *Audiology and Neurootology, 15*(6):399-406, 2010.

Timmer, F.C., Zhou, G., Guinan, J.J., Kujawa, S.G., Herrmann, B.S. and Rauch, S.D. "Vestibular evoked myogenic potential (VEMP) in patients with Ménière's disease with drop attacks." *Laryngoscope,116*(5):776-779, 2006.

Tumarkin, A. "The otolithic catastrophe: a new syndrome." *British Medical Journal, 25*(3942):175-177, 1936.

Viana, L.M., Bahmad. F. and Rauch, S.D. "Intratympanic gentamicin as a treatment for drop attacks in patients with Meniere's disease." *Laryngoscope,* 124(9):2151-2154, 2014.

CHAPTER FOUR
PROGNOSIS/PROGRESSION

Will I get better? When?
Will I get worse? When?
Will it spread to my other ear?
How much hearing will I lose? Will I go deaf?
Does the tinnitus get better? Worse?
How many years before the attacks go away?
How will my balance be in a few years?
Will I become disabled? What will I do?

Unfortunately there are many more questions than answers in Ménière's disease. Accurate predictions can't be made about the future of any single person. In some people the disease stops just as mysteriously as it began. For others the disorder and its effects stay their entire lives. Predictions are not only difficult because the disorder is so fickle but also because there have been no large studies looking at the disorder over a full life span.

Ménière's disease affects both the cochlea and vestibular areas of the inner ear. Measuring the progression of hearing loss is easiest because it can be measured accurately and objectively. The progression of vertigo and balance are more difficult to follow. There isn't general agreement on how to even measure vertigo/balance.

Prognosis/progression factoids:
- 60 to 80% of people get better or "stabilize on medical treatment" and do not require surgery or destruction of the inner ear.

- "Although episodes of vertigo that last longer than 6 hours are less frequent than shorter episodes, they occur with similar frequency throughout the natural course of the disease."

- More episodes of vertigo occur early in the disorder.

- If 12 months go by without an attack chances are 70% there won't be any over the following 12 months.

- 40% of the total number of people with Ménière's disease consider themselves to be disabled.

- Most of the hearing and vestibular losses occur over the first 5-10 years of the disorder.

- The chance Ménière's disease will affect the second ear increases as the years with Ménière's Disease increases and is between 12 and 83.7%, see table for more.

STUDY	NUMBER IN STUDY	YEARS STUDIED	BOTH EARS AFFECTED
Green	119	14	45%
Tokumanu			
"	243	10	12%
"	28	20	43%
Huppert	46	10	35%
		20	47%
Wladkowsky			34%
Gonzalez	225	5	83.7%
Sumi	29	10+	20.7%

- Constant illusion of motion: A study of 243 people found the percentage rose from 0-4% in people with Ménière's for 5 months to 21% in people who have had the disease for 20 years.

- 10 years into the disorder many people are missing 40 to 70 decibels of their hearing. While this is not complete deafness it does not allow an ear to hear an average human voice or use the telephone.

- The hearing loss commonly affects lower pitched sounds the most. The hearing loss in people with bilateral disease may be more extensive in each ear.

- Severe attacks can occur even 20 years into the disease.

- Elderly people with chronic dizziness/imbalance fall 2-3 times more than others.

- The condition generally burns itself out after 5-15 years and the episodes of vertigo cease, but there is a constant mild disequilibrium, tinnitus and moderate (not complete) unilateral hearing loss."
- Tokumasu found 5 out of 28 people had 10 or more attacks 10 years after the very first attack.

- A Finnish study of 183 people found 92% had permanent tinnitus, 19% of these people felt tinnitus was their most severe Ménière's disease symptom.

- Another Finnish study found that 68% of their subjects still had aural fullness after 16 years with Ménière's.

QUALITY OF LIFE

Trying to determine how bad life will become is difficult. In addition there is no standardized and easily measurable way, in widespread use, to measure misery, vestibular disability, social difficulties such as job loss or change, divorce, or relationship changes that can occur.

Bottom line, nobody can tell you what's ahead with any certainty. Some of the reasons for this:
- You might not have Ménière's disease.

- Each person responds differently to treatments.

- Various doctors have different approaches to treatment.

- The degree of turmoil caused depends a lot on a person's lifestyle and circumstances. For example, a young mountain climber would be more impacted than a less active retiree.

REFERENCES:

Ballester, M., Liard, P., Vibert, D. and Hausler, R. "Ménière's disease in the elderly." *Otology and Neurotology*, 23(1):73-78, 2002.

Belinchon, A., Perez-Garrigues, H., Tenias, J.M. and Lopez, A. "Hearing assessment in Ménière's disease." *The Laryngoscope, 121*:622-636, 2011.

Clemens, C. and Ruckenstein, M. "Characteristics of patients with unilateral and bilateral Ménière's disease." *Otology and Neurotology*, 33(7):1266-1269, 2012.

Gonzalez, M., Gonzalez, C., Trinidad, F.M., Ibanez, A., Pinilla, A., Martinez, M. Ruiz-Coello, A., Rodriguez Valiente, A. and Lopez-Cortijo C. "Medical management of Ménière's disease: A 10-year case series and review of literature." *European Archives of Otorhinolaryngology, 267*(9):1371-1376, 2010.

Green, J.D., Blum, D.J. and Harner, S.G. "Longitudinal followup of patients with Ménière's disease." *Otolaryngology-Head and Neck Surgery, 104*(6):783-788, 1991.

Havia, M. and Kentala, E. "Progression of symptoms of dizziness in Ménière's disease." *Archives of Otolaryngology-Head and Neck Surgery, 130*(4):431-435, 2004.

Huppert, D., Strupp, M. and Brandt, T. "Long-term course of Menière's disease revisited." *Acta Otolaryngology, 130*(6):644-651, 2010.

Ko, C., Hoffman, H. and Sklare, D.A. "Chronic imbalance or dizziness and falling: results from the 1994 disability supplement to the National Health interview survey and the second supplement on aging study." ARO meeting, Abstract 470, 2006.

Levo, H., Kentala, E., Rasku, J. and Pyykkö, I. "Aural fullness in Ménière's disease." *Audiology and Neurootology, 19*(6):395-399, 2014.

Perez, R., Chen, J.M. and Nedzelski, J.M. "The status of the contralateral ear in established unilateral Meniere's disease." *Laryngoscope, 114*(8):1373-1376, 2004.

Savastano, M., Guerrieri, V. and Marioni, G. "Evolution of audiometric pattern in Ménière's disease: long-term survey of 380 cases evaluated according to the 1995 guidelines of the American Academy of Otolaryngology-head and neck surgery." *Journal of Otolaryngology, 35*(1):26-29, 2006.

Sato, G., Sekine, K., Matsuda, K., Ueeda, H., Horii, A., Nishiike, S., Kitahara, T., Uno, A., Imai, T., Inohara, H. and Takeda, N. "Long-term prognosis of hearing loss in patients with unilateral Ménière's disease." *Acta Otolaryngologica, 134*(10):1005-1010, 2014.

Sumi, T., Watanabe, I., Tsunoda, A., Nishio, A., Komatsuzaki, A. and Kitamura, K. "Longitudinal study of 29 patients with Meniere's disease with follow-up of 10 years or more." *Acta Oto-Laryngologica, 132*:10-15. 2012.

Tokumasu, K., Fujino, A., Naganuma, H., Hoshino, I. and Arai, M. "Initial symptoms and restrospective evaluation of prognosis in Ménière's disease." *Acta Otolaryngologica Supplement, 524*:43-49, 1996.

Yoshida, T., Stephens, D., Kentala, E., Levo, H., Auramo, Y., Poe, D. and Pyykko, I. "Tinnitus complaint behavior in long-standing Ménière's disorder: its association with the other cardinal symptoms." *Clinical Otolaryngology,* 36:461-467, 2011.

SECTION II
IN DEPTH

CHAPTER FIVE
STRESS

Dry mouth, goose bumps, cold sweat, racing heart, hyperventilation, anxiety, worry, fear, trembling and more, can all be part of the Ménière's experience. These are also signs of the body's response to stress.

> Stress is any event or situation interfering with the normal physical and/or mental/emotional function of the body. It's the confrontation with more than we can physically or mentally handle.

The immediate effect of a large threat is the release of the catecholamine chemicals, including adrenaline, throughout the body by the autonomic nervous system. This chemical release quickly prepares us for a "fight or flight" response by increasing heart rate and blood pressure, releasing glucose into the blood stream, slowing digestion, dilating muscle blood vessels, dilating the pupils, relaxing the bladder, and making us much more alert. Dry mouth, trembling, and the rest, are also the result of this response.

This is an excellent response if being chased through the woods by a bear but not helpful during a Ménière's attack when neither fighting nor fleeing are helpful or possible.

Ménière's disease can cause a "fight or flight" response in at least two ways. It can be produced by our emotional/mental response to the Ménière's and through the vestibular autonomic reflexes.

Stress affects our inner ears in a number of ways:
- Increases endolymph leading to an increase in the number of symptoms and/or their intensity.

- Sodium and water retention leads to increased fluid pressure around the brain. This increased pressure can cause symptoms by disturbing the damaged areas of the inner ear.

- Elevated blood sugar levels lead to increased inner ear fluids. If the blood sugar level fluctuates, the symptoms can increase and decrease in severity as well.

- Increased fatty acid levels can lead to cholesterol deposits in blood vessels including those supplying the ear. Blood flow to these areas could be slowed down or even stopped.

- The possibility also exists that increased levels of steroids and/or adrenaline right in the inner ear may also lead to physical changes and symptoms.

- Compensation, in people who already have a partial loss of vestibular function, can begin to unravel under stress.

These symptoms can plague people between attacks and might even be produced by thinking about an attack. A lower level of stress can also exist without being noticed.

Stress continuing for long periods of time takes a toll on the body with wide ranging problems including:
- Salt and water retention leading to increased blood volume and blood pressure.

- Stress can also lead to behaviour that in turn causes vestibular problems. Drinking alcohol, having too much caffeine (coffee, chocolate), eating too many refined carbohydrates (candy, cookies, bread, and pasta) and overeating salt can cause Ménière's symptoms in some people.

- Increased appetite.

- Excessive amounts of steroids and adrenaline in the blood stream can compromise the immune system.

- Increased blood sugar level.

- Increased fatty acid levels leading to increased cholesterol.

- Decreased melatonin leading to insomnia.

- Feelings of anxiety, hopelessness and impending doom.

- Errors in judgment and memory loss.

- Ménière's is stressful and may set up a never ending cycle of stress worsening the Ménière's which in turn increases the stress level in a never ending cycle.

Stress cuts both ways in Ménière's disease. Ménière's disease definitely causes stress and stress has always been named as a factor causing Ménière's disease or at least bringing on its attacks. Research has found elevated stress hormones in people with Ménière's disease and has determined the inner ear is affected by it. Evidence that Ménière's disease can lead to the symptoms of post-traumatic stress disorder (PTSD) has been found as well.

A person can try to ignore stress, attempt to remove it from their life, do things that reduce the stress or it's effects, use stress to their advantage (when possible), rethink how they look at stressful situations and events, seek treatment for the problems and symptoms stress has created, and/or undergo counselling or therapy to improve their situation.

Day to day stress is a part of the human condition. Removing all of it and still being a part of the world isn't a realistic possibility. The issue isn't so much if we have stress, but how we handle, treat or use the stress we have. Simply ignoring stress works for some people but for others this approach spells trouble. The long-term effects of stress can be just too serious to ignore. Removing all stress sounds good in theory but in reality a person would just about have to leave the world, as they knew it, and crawl into a cave to be free of the stresses of modern life.

The effects of stress can be limited by a number of approaches including just plain getting out and having some fun, a good program of exercise for about 30 minutes three times each week, yoga, relaxation therapy, listening to music, setting aside time to relax, getting enough sleep, guided imagery, hobbies and talking about stressful situations with people who understand. In some situations drug therapy may also be suggested and is safest when an experienced therapist is directing the care and writing the prescriptions.

Some research findings suggest uncertainty stresses many people with Ménière's disease. People are stressed by the uncertainty of what causes the disorder, how it can be treated, when the next attack will occur, how bad will it be, how much damage is going to occur, how people feel about them, what to do and the list goes on. Ménière's certainly breeds uncertainty on many levels.

Stress is a part of the human condition and for most people it's also a part of Ménière's disease. Some steps can be taken to reduce it, see more in Chapter 30, "Coping and Staying Safe," page 193.

REFERENCES:

Aoki, M., Yokota, Y., Hayashi, T., Kuze, B., Murai, M., Misuta, K. and Ito, Y. "Disorder of the saliva melatonin circadian rhythm in patients with Ménière's disease." *Acta Neurologica Scandanavia, 113*(4):256-261, 2006.

Falkenius-Schmidt, K., Rymarker, S. and Horner, K.C. "Hyperprolactinemia in some Ménière's patients even in the absence of incapacitating vertigo." *Hearing Research, 203*(102):154-158, 2005.

Guyton, A.C. and Hall, J.E. *Guyton and Hall Textbook of Medical Physiology.* 11th edition. Philadelphia: W.B. Saunders, 2010.

Horner, K.C. and Cazals, Y. "Stress in hearing and balance in Ménière's disease." *Noise and Health, 5(*20):29-34, 2003.

Horner, K.C. and Cazals, Y. "Stress hormones in Ménière's disease and acoustic neuroma." *Brain Research Bulletin, 66*(1):1-8, 2005.

Kirby, S.E. and Yardley, L. "The contribution of symptoms of posttraumatic stress disorder, health anxiety and intolerance of uncertainty to distress in Ménière's disease." *Journal of Nervous and Mental Disorders, 197*(5):324-329, 2009.

Kirby, S.E. and Yardley, L. "Cognitions associated with anxiety in Ménière's disease." *Journal of Psychosomatic Research, 66*(2):111-118, 2009.

Kirby, S.E. and Yardley, L. "Understanding psychological distress in Ménière's disease: A systematic review" *Psychology, Health & Medicine, 13*(3):257-273, 2008.

Marieb, E.N. and Hoehn, K. *Human Anatomy and Physiology, 9th edition.* London:Pearson, 2012.

Orji, F. "The Influence of Psychological Factors in Ménière's Disease." *Annals of Medical and Health Sciences Research, 4*(1):3-7, 2014.

Sobrinho, L.G. "Prolactin, psychological stress and environment in humans: Adaptation and maladaptation." *Pituitary, 6*(1):35-39, 2003.

Söderman, A.C., Möller, J., Bagger-Sjöbäck, D., Bergenius, J. and Hallqvist, J. "Stress as a trigger of attacks in Menière's disease. A case-crossover study." *Laryngoscope, 114*(10):1843-1848, 2004.

Van Cruijsen, N., Dullaart, R.P., Wit, H.P. and Albers, F.W. "Analysis of cortisol and other stress related hormones in patients with Ménière's disease." *Otology and Neurotology, 26*(6):1214-1219, 2005.

Yates, B.J. and Bronstein, A.M. "The effects of vestibular system lesions on autonomic regulation: Observations, mechanisms, and clinical implications." *Journal of Vestibular Research, 15:*119-129, 2005.

CHAPTER SIX
ADJUSTMENT/COMPENSATION

Life with Ménière's disease is all about adjustment. Intellectual adjustment to the new physical, social and emotional realities, to the new reality of chronic illness, to the loss and upheaval as well as to the changed rhythm of life can be nearly continual.

The most important adjustment is a physical one done behind the scenes in the brain. How the brain adjusts depends upon many factors:

- One ear or both ears: A loss in one ear is easier to adjust to than loss in both.

- Permanent loss or fluctuating: A permanent loss is easier to adjust to than fluctuating levels of function. Attacks closer together than 2-3 months can prevent the brain from adjusting.

- Types of drugs being taken: Alcohol, antimotion sickness drugs, antinausea drugs and sedatives all interfere with the brain's adjustment process.

- Activity level: The more physical activity the better.

The adjustment process for loss on one side is called vestibular compensation. When both sides have been lost the process is called sensory substitution.

COMPENSATION

When a partial loss of vestibular function occurs, the brain immediately begins the natural process of vestibular compensation. This allows the brain to readjust how it interprets vestibular information by relying upon the information coming from just one ear. Therapy can be aimed at helping this along a bit by encouraging the use of vision and movement, two activities crucial for vestibular compensation.

A partial loss includes any of the following situations:
- Reduced information from one ear.

- Reduced information from both ears.

- No information at all from one ear.

- No information at all from one ear and reduced information from the other.

The term vestibular compensation refers specifically to the chemical changes that occur in the brain allowing it to continue carrying out its balance function after a partial vestibular loss.

Compensation is not a static situation. It can be undone or decreased by further attacks, stress, illness, and alcohol as well as drugs affecting the brain. Muscle relaxants, painkillers and general anesthesia all have a brain affect.

SENSORY SUBSTITUTION

If almost all the vestibular function is lost on both sides the brain must change from using three sensory systems to using two. It must come to rely only on vision and proprioception, in essence to substitute these for the lost vestibular sense. Over time with practice and experience balance will improve and symptoms will lessen. The medical term for this process is sensory substitution.

Sometimes sensory substitution occurs when it shouldn't, when vestibular information is not gone. It can be the cause of symptoms rather than a mechanism to reduce them. Physical therapy can help retrain the brain to use the appropriate amounts of information from the various sensory systems.

HELPING COMPENSATION AND SENSORY SUBSTITUTION

What you can do:

- After an attack get up and about as soon as possible and SAFE. Open and use your eyes as soon as possible. Move your head around freely, don't hold it stiffly.

- Exercise daily by walking and moving your head, arms and legs. More vigorous exercise is even better if you are able to do so safely.

- Abstain from alcohol and any other drugs that affect brain function.

- Stop taking anti-symptom drugs such as Valium, Xanax, Dramamine, Antivert, etc. as soon as possible after an attack.

- Get enough rest and sleep, eat a healthy diet.

Physical therapy (vestibular rehabilitation) with vision and movement exercises can be very helpful for some people, particularly when delivered by a physical therapist with education and experience in vestibular disorders and Ménière's disease. This will not stop whatever is causing the Ménière's disease but can help with many of the symptoms that surround it.

REFERENCES:

Balaban, C.D., Hoffer, M.E and Gottshall, K.R. "Top-down approach to vestibular compensation: Translational lessons from vestibular rehabilitation." *Brain Research, 1482*:101-111, 2012.

Cawthorne, T.E. "The physiological basis for head exercises." *Journal of the Chartered Society of Physiotherapy, 29*:106, 1944.

Cawthorne, T. "Vestibular injuries." *Proceedings of the Royal Society of Medicine, 39*:270-272, 1945.

Gottshall, K.R., Topp, S.G. and Hoffer, M.E. "Early vestibular physical therapy rehabilitation for Meniere's disease." *Otolaryngological Clinics of North America, 43*(5):1113-1119, 2010.

Hain, T.C., Fuller, L., Weil, L., and Kotsias, J. "Effects of T'ai Chi on Balance." *Archives of Otolaryngology-Head and Neck Surgery, 125*(11):1191-1195, 1999.

Herdman, S.J. and Clendaniel, R. *Vestibular Rehabilitation,* 4th edition. Philadelphia: F.A. Davis Company, 2014.

Horak, F.B. "Postural compensation for vestibular loss and implications for rehabilitation." *Restorative Neurology and Neuroscience, 28*(1):57-68, 2010.

McCabe, B.F. "Labyrinthine exercises in the treatment of diseases characterized by vertigo: their physiologic basis and methodology." *Laryngoscope, 80*:1429, 1970.

CHAPTER SEVEN
LIFE EFFECT, QUALITY OF LIFE

Ménière's disease can change life in many ways, well beyond the physical. Social skills, relationships, a person's view of themselves, the way others view them as well as their place in society change. This disorder can become the entire focus of life, always on the mind and impacting every decision and very nearly every thought. The quality of life is decreased in many people with Ménière's disease.

A person's journey through life is usually made without thinking about illness or personal mortality, until something like Ménière's disease strikes. This disorder stops any thoughts of invincibility or that bad things only happen to other people. It can bring a protective wall of denial crashing down leaving uncertainty, insecurity, doubt, confusion and fear in its place.

This disorder can create feelings of uncertainty, anxiety, being bad, degradation, doubt, dread, embarrassment in front of others, exhaustion, failure, feeling of being handicapped, frustration, guilt, impending catastrophe, inferiority, insecurity, loneliness, loss of control, loss of dignity, rejection, sadness, shame, self-blame, sleep disturbances, social isolation, terror, and more. One study found the only disorders more intrusive were fibromyalgia, anxiety disorder and HIV AIDS. Another study of 484 people with Ménière's disease found more than half were experiencing partial or full symptoms of PTSD, post-traumatic stress disorder.

It's thought that the uncertainty of Ménière's disease is a major cause of anxiety. In addition to anxiety many people experience depressed feelings. One study found 35.5% of people with inactive disease were affected as well as 71% with active disease. A German study found that men suffer from a slighter higher level of depression and anxiety.

Also causing anxiety is the intolerance of uncertainty, fear/avoidance of physical activity and a belief that dizziness will always turn into a severe attack of vertigo.

Not surprisingly studies have found that increased symptoms lead to decreased quality of life, good social supports increase quality of life and negative coping, such as the use of illegal drugs, lead to a decreased quality of life.

Even the most intimate parts of life are not spared. One study looking at sexual practices found many men with Ménière's disease had experienced erectile dysfunction and that some woman experienced less sexual desire.

In addition, the lives of the partners, relatives and friends of people with Ménière's disease are also impacted. Their focus is also on the uncertainty of life and the restrictions the disease has now put on them. Significantly, one piece of research has found that these people tend to focus on the symptoms rather than lifestyle and quality of life effects.

A transformation from "normal" person to sick person may take place. In the 1950's the sociologist Parsons first described a societal role change he called the "sick role." According to Parsons a person taking on the sick role is excused from performing normal roles and duties and society does not find them responsible for their situation. In return society expects sick people to want to get well and work actively to get there by using competent health care professionals.

In the short term the sick role is acceptable to society but as time goes by the situation changes. Ménière's disease victims may find themselves being blamed for their situation by friends, coworkers and relatives and even health care professionals. These people may believe not enough has been done to rid the victim of the disorder or, worse, somehow a sick person likes having the disorder and the sick role.

Patients expect to be met with understanding, sympathy and competence, to have their problems affirmed and to be helped. Instead, over time a doctor may come to blame the patient for their Ménière's disease, particularly if they feel powerless to stop the suffering or disease progression. Blaming the victim means the doctor doesn't have to feel responsible for failing to successfully treat this chronic disorder. It can also signal a doctor is not actively looking into all the different treatments available. They may also feel their patient is overusing the sick role and receiving "secondary gain" from their situation, i.e. that they like the attention received while sick or perhaps like getting sick pay and not working.

Friends and acquaintances may stop calling or coming around. Some won't know how to interact with an ill person. Others turn away because they can't tolerate the notion their friend or colleague is suffering.

Some will feel emotionally threatened by the illness and hide from it as best they can. They may also stop coming because they miss their old friend and might not like the new one who has taken their place. On the other hand, in a study looking for positive experiences associated with Ménière's disease, participants mentioned finding new friends, with the disorder, as a positive.

It's easy to feel threatened by Ménière's disease. Life's events are often random and beyond human control. Some people choose to ignore this randomness and believe they are in control, the masters of their own fate. They believe their actions and behavior keep them well, that they owe nothing to luck or chance. To accept that Ménière's disease is random and can't be controlled is to accept that all humans are vulnerable, all at risk, that anyone can get "it." Some people find it less intimidating to feel the victim's actions or lack of action are the "real" problem and blame the victims for their illness.

Ménière's disease may also stop a person from maturing and evolving emotionally. There are a number of theories explaining how humans mature through life. Looking at one theory, Maslow's Hierarchy of Needs, can help understand some of the symptoms and life changes brought by Ménière's disease.

Maslow described five basic needs throughout life, physiologic/survival, safety/security, loving/belonging, self-esteem and self-actualization, arranged in a pyramid with physiologic/survival on the bottom and self-actualization at the top. Each need must be fulfilled before climbing up to the next.

Physiologic/survival is the first and most basic need for air, food, and water. Attacks of violent vertigo can interfere with this most basic of needs. Having the need unfulfilled causes life to become all about trying to stop the attacks, take care of one's self, to drink, to eat. Once the need is met, life is no longer focused exclusively on this basic struggle for survival.

The next need on the pyramid is safety/security. Without the feeling of safety and security life is filled with apprehension, fear, tension, anxiety, dread, nervousness and a feeling of lost control fills life. Safety/security needs are hard to meet when suffering violent attacks of vertigo   at irregular   intervals, experiencing   hearing   loss   and/or impaired vision, having decreased ability to think and remember as well as difficulty walking and getting around. When this need is met one feels safe, calm, relaxed; restful sleep, learning, remembering, thinking, perception and attentiveness are possible once again.

After the physiologic/survival and safety/security needs have been met loving/belonging becomes important. If loving/belonging go unmet loneliness, rejection, friendlessness and rootlessness are experienced. Ménière's can interfere with this due to the trouble reading and writing, discomfort from loud noise, the hungover/fatigue feeling, fear of leaving home and poor memory that force a withdrawal from normal interaction with co-workers, friends, and relatives. When the need is met a person feels loved, has the feeling of a place in society, and is able to love.

To feel self-reliant, self-confident, and competent as well as experience achievement in life the need for self-esteem must be met. This can only be met if a person is independent and engaging in their usual activities. When this need goes unmet there are feelings of inferiority, weakness, helplessness and discouragement.

The last and highest need is self-actualization. It can't be met until those below it have been fulfilled. If this need goes unmet mental restlessness results; when it is met a person can be productive in their life.

Sadly, attacks of Ménière's disease interfere with meeting all needs from the most basic right up to the most advanced. This can lead to total fixation on the Ménière's disease and feeling fearful, tense, nervous, misunderstood, unloved, inferior, helpless, discouraged and non-productive.

How much life is impacted by Ménière's disease depends upon a complex web of factors. The number and severity of Ménière's symptoms, physical, emotional, and intellectual abilities, prior history and experience with illness, as well as how colleagues, friends, neighbors, relatives and doctors respond to the disorder all play a part. Understanding your reactions to, and feelings about, Ménière's disease as well as those of the people around you may help in understanding how and why life has changed and how to deal with it.

Ménière's disease need not be totally bad. People with the disorder make new friends, become better able to listen to their "inner voice," set more realistic goals and become better people at work because they are more cooperative and better able to delegate responsibility, according to one study looking at the positive effects of the disorder.

The old adage, "life is what you make of it" still applies in Ménière's disease. Even if life has been turned upside down it can still go on in some form with some work.

REFERENCES:

Arroll, M., Dancey, C.P., Attree, E.A., Smith, S. and James, T. "People with symptoms of Ménière's disease: The relationship between illness intrusiveness, illness uncertainty, dizziness handicap and depression." *Otology and Neurotology*, *33*(5):816-823, 2012.

Christopoulos, K.A. "The sick role in literature and society." *JAMA*, *285*:93, 2001.

Coker, N.J., Coker, R.R., Jenkins, H.A. and Vincent, K.R. "Psychological profile of patients with Ménière's disease." *Archives of Otolaryngology-Head and Neck Surgery*, *115*:1355-1357, 1989.

Duracinsky, M., Mosnier, I., Bouccara, D., Sterkers, O. and Chassany, O. "Working Group of the Societe Francaise, d'Otorhinolaryngologie (ORL)." *Value Health*, *10*(4):273-284, 2007.

Erlandsson, S.I., Eriksson-Mangold, M. and Wiberg, A. "Meniere's disease: Trauma, distress and adaptation studied through focus interview analyses." *Scandinavian Audiology*, *25*(Supp 43):45-55, 1996.

Haybach, P.J. "Maslow's Hierarchy of needs and the individual with chronic vestibular dysfunction." *ORL Head and Neck Nursing*, *12*(2):14-17, 1994.

Holgers, K. and Finizia, C. "Health profiles for patient with Ménière's Disease." 2001 [cited 2013 January 25]; 4:71:80 Available from http//www.noiseand health.org/text.asp?2001/4/13/71/31801

Kirby, S.E. and Yardley, L. "Conditions associated with anxiety in Ménière's Disease." *Journal of Psychosomatic Research*, *66*(2):111-118, 2004.

Kirby, S.E. and Yardley, L. "The contribution of symptoms of posttraumatic stress disorder, health anxiety and intolerance of uncertainty to distress in Ménière's disease." *Journal of Nervous and Mental Disease*, *197*(5):324-329, 2009.

Kurre, A., Strauman, D., Van Gool, C.A., Gloor-Juzi, T. and Bastiaenen, C. "Gender differences in patients with dizziness and unsteadiness regarding self-perceived disability, anxiety, depression, and its associations." *BioMedCentral Ear, Nose and Throat Disorders*, *12*:1-12, 2012.

Levo, H., Stephens, D., Poe, D., Kentala, E. and Pyykko, I. "Use of ICF in assessing the effects of Ménière's Disease on life. " *Annals of Otology Rhinology Laryngology*, *119*(9):583-589, 2010.

Lopez-Escamez, J.A., Viciana, D. and Garrido-Fernandez, P. "Impact of bilaterality and headache on health-related quality of life in Ménière's Disease." *Annals of Otology, Rhinology and Laryngology*, *118*(6):409-416, 2009.

Maslow, A.H. *Motivation and Personality.* New York: Harper & Row, 1954.

Maslow, A.H. *Motivation and Personality.* New York: Harper & Row, 1970.

Mendel, B., Lutzen, K., Bergenius, J. and Bjorvell, H. "Living with dizziness: an explorative study." *Journal of Advanced Nursing*, *26:*1134-1141, 1997.

Nakayama, M., Suzuki, M., Inagaki, A., Takemura, L., Watanabe, N., Tanigawa, T., Okamoto, K., Hattori, H., Brodie, H. and Murakami., S. "Impaired quality of sleep in Ménière's disease patients." *Journal of Clinical Sleep Medicine," 6*(5):445-449, 2010.

Orji, F.T. "Influence of psychological factors in Meniere's disease." *Annals of Medical Health Science Reseasrch*, *4*(1): 3–7, 2014.

Parsons, T. *The Social System*. Glencoe, IL: The Free Press, 1951.

Porter, M. and Boothroyd, R.A. "Symptom severity, social supports, coping styles and quality of life among individuals diagnosed with Ménière's Disease." *Chronic Illness*, *11*(4):256-266, 2015.

Pyykkő, I., Manchaiah, V., Levo, H., Kentala, E. and Rasku, J. "Attitudes of significant others of people with Ménière's disease vary from coping to victimization." *International Journal of Audiology, 54*(5):316-22, 2015.

Stephens, D., Kentala, E., Varpa, K. and Pyykko, I. "Positive experiences associated with Ménière's disorder." *Otology & Neurotology*, *28*:982-987, 2007.

Stephens, D., Pyykko, I., Levo, H., Poe, D., Kentala, E. and Auramo, Y. "Positive experiences and quality of life in Ménière's Disease." *International Journal of Audiology, 49*(11):839-843, 2010.

Stephens, D., Pyykko, I., Kentala, E., Levo, H. and Rasku, J. "The effects of Meniere's disease on the patients significant others." *International Journal of Audiology, 51*(12):858-863, 2012.

Yardley, L. *Vertigo and Dizziness*. New York: Routledge, 1994.

Zapata, C. and Lopez-Eccamez, J.A. "A pilot study of sexual health practices in patients with Ménière's disease." *Acta Otorrinolaringologia, 62*(2):119-125, 2011.

CHAPTER EIGHT
VISION, EYES

There's a close relationship between the inner ears, the eyes and balance. Vision is needed for optimum balance and vestibular information from the inner ear is needed for optimum vision. A disruption in this relationship creates a number of Ménière's disease symptoms and is also the basis for many vestibular tests and treatment.

Vision is one of the three senses needed for the best balance to take place. The inner ears can't provide information about movement at a constant speed but vision can. When moving at a constant speed toward an object, the object gets bigger and when moving away, smaller. It also provides information about a person's movement or position in relationship to their surroundings.

Vestibular information is needed to keep vision clear and useful while moving around or moving the head. This is done through two different reflexes, the VOR and the VCR.

Of the three systems involved in balance, vision is the one most easily fooled. A person can be tricked into thinking they are moving when they aren't and into thinking they aren't when they are. Have you ever stepped on your brakes while sitting still because the car next to you moved? That's your vision fooling you. Vision will also tell a person they aren't moving when in a windowless room on board a ship even when the seas are rough. When the visual information doesn't match with the proprioceptive and vestibular information motion sickness can result.

Problems with glare and the flicker of fluorescent lighting, reading, eye jerking (nystagmus) and bouncing vision called oscillopsia are all possible in Ménière's disease as well as trouble watching movement or walking in visually stimulating environments like a supermarket, fabric store, or an airport. Watching movement can also lead to motion sickness and imbalance.

HOW OR WHY ARE THESE A PROBLEM?
- *Flickering light* may be perceived as body movement which conflicts with other information being received by the brain leading to discomfort and possibly motion sickness.

- *Trouble reading* can come from problems with thought and memory and/or jerking movement of the eyes that make it difficult to follow a line of print.

- *Supermarkets* and other visually stimulating places give the illusion of movement and may not provide a steady visual reference of where horizontal is.

- *Watching movement* may convince the brain that movement is occurring when it isn't. This will conflict with both vestibular and proprioceptive information.

In the aftermath of an attack or in the later stages of the disease there may be an increased dependence upon vision. This can include the need to see the feet while walking. People wearing progressive, trifocal, and bifocal glasses may have trouble because these lenses distort vision when looking down. They can potentially lead to motion sickness and imbalance as well.

It's also possible for the brain to depend abnormally upon vision and not enough on vestibular information. Symptoms like motion sickness can occur when watching a moving object, particularly large ones like the movement on a movie screen, in malls and supermarkets, crowds, traffic, looking up at the clouds in the sky. A physical therapy evaluation by a therapist experienced in dealing with vestibular disorders can determine if someone is leaning too heavily on vision for their balance and then prescribe exercises to decrease this dependence.

The opposite can also occur, a person may have difficulty adjusting to a loss of vestibular function and fail to depend more upon vision. This, too, may be helped by physical therapy.

Vision case report: There has been one report of someone with Ménière's disease having difficulty after a multifocal intraocular lens implantation. Before having eye surgery discuss your situation with your eye surgeon.

REFERENCES:

Bronstein, A. M. "Vision and vertigo: some visual aspects of vestibular disorders." *Journal of Neurology, 251*(4):381-387, 2004.

Herdman, S.J. and Clendaniel, R. *Vestibular Rehabilitation,* 4th edition. Philadelphia: F.A. Davis Company, 2014.

Leigh, R.J. and Zee, D.S. *The Neurology of Eye Movements,* 4th edition, USA: Oxford University Press, 2006.

Gatzioufas, Z., Osvald, A., Schroeder, A.C, Kozeis, N. and Seitz, B. "A serious refractive multifocal intraocular lens complication in Meniere's disease." *Optometry and Vision Science, 87*(6):448-449, 2010.

CHAPTER NINE
THOUGHT, MEMORY, PERCEPTION OF SELF

Complaints from people with Ménière's disease and other vestibular disorders about difficulty with short-term memory, thought and math as well as feeling disconnected or not in their own body are nothing new, but in the past there was little scientific evidence to show a relationship between vestibular dysfunction and these problems. As a result some people were considered to be "nut cases" when they tried to discuss these problems with health care professionals. There were even studies in the past seemingly trying to portray Ménière's disease as a psychiatric disorder because of some of these complaints.

Some researchers and others were listening. Over the last twenty years a body of research showing a vestibular effect on thought and memory as well as a thought and memory effect on vestibular function and balance has developed and grown. It's also now thought, "vestibular signals contribute to the experience that the self is located within the boundaries of the body." So, if the vestibular signals are absent or changed the feeling of the self not being within the boundaries of the body would be possible.

In January 2016 the online journal *Frontiers in Integrative Neuroscience* made "The Vestibular System in Cognitive and Memory Processes in Mammals" freely available online as a PDF ebook. (journal.frontiersin.org/researchtopic/1235/the-vestibular-system-in-cognitive-and-memory-processes-in-mammalians). It contains a number of articles about this area of study.

Although it's a free online source this journal contains very scientific, scholarly articles by researchers and is best understood by people working in this field. There are some bits and pieces the average reader will find informational.

In short, when the brain has to make a choice between balance and thought, it chooses balance. Because the brain is receiving vestibular, visual and proprioceptive information there's less ability left to work on thought. Balance activities also use cognition, leaving even less cognitive ability for other activities needing it.

To make matters worse thought and memory can also be affected by the stress and anxiety of this unpredictable disorder. The very medications given to relieve the vertigo, nausea and vomiting can also contribute to the problem.

The 2008 U.S. National Health survey found people with vestibular vertigo had an:

- Eightfold increased odds of serious difficulty concentrating or remembering.

- Fourfold increased odds of activity limitation due to difficulty remembering or confusion.

- Threefold increased odds of depression, anxiety and panic disorder.

TREATMENT

The focus of research has been on the basic relationship between thought, memory, the vestibular system and balance. This has raised the possibility of a future drug treatment to improve the situation.

Thought and memory issues should be discussed carefully with a physician to make sure there isn't a treatable cause such as the drugs in use or some physical change like dehydration or another disease altogether.

Drugs are used to improve thought and/or memory in dyslexia (Piracetam) and ADD/ADHD (Strattera). There are claims some diet supplements and foods such as black tea and green tea can help thought and memory. None of these have been studied in people with vestibular disorders. We don't know if they are helpful or if they might even be harmful to someone with Ménière's disease.

SUM UP

Tasks requiring thought take longer to carry out and are less accurate when the vestibular system is being taxed. On the flip side mental tasks can decrease balance ability.

The "The Living On" chapter has some suggestions for helping with thinking and making decisions.

REFERENCES:

Andersson, G., Hagman, J., Talianzadeh, R., Svedberg, A. and Larsen, H.C. "Dual-task study of cognitive and postural interference in patients with vestibular disorders." *Otology and Neurotology, 24*(2):289-293, 2003.

Andersson, G., Hagman, J., Talianzadeh, R., Svedberg, A. and Larsen, H.C. "Effect of cognitive load on postural control." *Brain Research Bulletin, 58*(1):135-139, 2002.

Andersson, G., Yardley, L. and Luxon, L. "A dual-task study of interference between mental activity and control of balance." *American Journal of Otology, 19*(5):632-637, 1998.

Barra, J., Bray, A., Sahni, V., Golding, J.F. and Gresty, M.A. "Increasing cognitive load with increasing balance challenge: recipe for catastrophe." *Experimental Brain Research, 174*(4):734-745, 2006.

Bigelow, R.T., Semenov, Y.R., du Lac, S., Hoffman, H.J. and Agrawal, Y. "Vestibular vertigo and comorbid cognitive and psychiatric impairment: the 2008 National Health Interview Survey." *Journal of Neurology and Neurosurgery and Psychiatry,* doi:10.1136/jnnp-2015-310319

Brandt, T., Schautzer, F., Hamilton, D.A., Brüning, R., Markowitsch, H.J., Kalla, R., Darlington, C., Smith, P. and Strupp, M. "Vestibular loss causes hippocampal atrophy and impaired spatial memory in humans." *Brain, 128*(Pt 11):2732-2741, 2005.

Ehrenfried, T., Guerraz, M., Thilo, K.V., Yardley, L. and Gresty, M.A. "Posture and mental task performance when viewing a moving visual field." *Brain Research Cognitive Brain Research, 17*(1):140-153, 2003.

Grimm, R.J., Hemenway, W.G., Lebray, P.R., and Black, F.O. "The perilymph fistula syndrome defined in mild head trauma." *Acta otolaryngologica Supplement, 464*:1040, 1989.

Hanes, D.A. and McCollum, G. "Cognitive-vestibular interactions: A review of patient difficulties and possible mechanisms." *Journal of Vestibular Research, 16*(3):75-91, 2006.

Hitier, M., Besnard, S. and Smith, P.F. "Vestibular pathways involved in cognition." *Frontiers in Integrated Neuroscience, 23*;8:59. doi: 10.3389/fnint.2014.00059. eCollection 2014.

Hüfner, K., Hamilton, D.A., Kalla, R., Stephan, T., Glasauer, S., Ma, J., Brüning, R., Markowitsch, H.J., Labudda, K., Schichor, C., Strupp, M. and Brandt, T. "Spatial memory and hippocampal volume in humans with unilateral vestibular deafferentation." *Hippocampus, 17*(6):471-485, 2007.

Kirby, S.E. and Yardley, L. "Cognitions associated with anxiety in Ménière's disease." *Journal of Psychosomatic Research, 66*(2):111-118, 2009.

Marieb, E.N. and Hoehn, K. "Human Anatomy and Physiology," 9th ed N.J.:Pearson. 2012.

Pellecchia, G.L. "Postural sway increases with attentional demands of concurrent cognitive task." *Gait Posture, 18*(1):29-34, 2003.

Quant, S., Adkin, A.L., Staines, W.R. and McIlroy, W.E. "Cortical activation following a balance disturbance." *Experimental Brain Research, 155*(3):393-400, 2004.

Rankin, J.K., Woollacott, M.H., Shumway-Cook, A. and Brown, L.A. "Cognitive influence on postural stability: a neuromuscular analysis in young and older adults." *Journal of Gerontology and Biological Science and Medical Science*, *55*(3):M112-9, 2000.

Redfern, M.S., Talkowski, M.E., Jennings, J.R. and Furman, J.M. "Cognitive influences in postural control of patients with unilateral vestibular loss." *Gait Posture*, *19*(2):105-114, 2004.

Riley, M.A., Baker, A.A., and Schmit, J.M. "Inverse relation between postural variability and difficulty of a concurrent short-term memory task." *Brain Research Bulletin*, *62*(3):191-195, 2003.

Risey, J. and Briner, W. "Dyscalculia in patients with vertigo." *Journal of Vestibular Research, 1*:31-37, 1990.

Schautzer, F., Hamilton, D., Kalla, R., Strupp, M. and Brandt, T. "Spatial memory deficits in patients with chronic bilateral vestibular failure." *Annals of the New York Academy of Science, 1004*:316-324, 2003.

Shumway-Cook, A. and Woollacott, M. "Attentional demands and postural control: the effect of sensory context." *Journal of Gerontology. Series A, Biological Sciences and Medical Sciences, 55*(1):M10-6, 2000.

Smith, P.F., Horii, A., Russell, N., Bilkey, D.K., Zheng, Y., Liu, P., Kerr, D.S. and Darlington, C.L. "The effects of vestibular lesions on hippocampal function in rats." *Progress in Neurobiology, 75(6)*:391-405, 2005.

Talkowski, M.E., Redfern, M.S., Jennings, J.R. and Furman, J.M. "Cognitive Requirements for Vestibular and Ocular Motor Processing in Healthy Adults and Patients with Unilateral Vestibular Lesions." *Journal of Cognitive Neuroscience, 17*:1432-1441, 2005.

Wallace, D.G., Hines, D.J., Pellis, S.M. and Whishaw, I.Q. "Vestibular information is required for dead reckoning in the rat." *Journal of Neuroscience, 22*(22):10009-10017, 2002.

Yardley, L., Papo, D., Bronstein, A., Gresty, M., Gardner, M., Lavie, N. and Luxon, L. "Attentional demands of continuously monitoring orientation using vestibular information." *Neuropsychologia, 40(4)*:373-83, 2002.

Yardley, L., Gardner, M., Bronstein, A., Davies, R., Buckwell, D. and Luxon, L. "Interference between postural control and mental task performance in patients with vestibular disorder and healthy controls." *Journal of Neurology, Neurosurgery and Psychiatry, 71*(1):48-52, 2001.

Yen, F., Sang, F., Jáuregui-Renaud, K., Green, D. A., Bronstein, A. M., and Gresty, M. A. "Depersonalisation / derealisation symptoms in vestibular disease." *Journal of Neurology Neurosurgery Psychiatry* 77:6 760-766, 2006.

Zheng, Y., Darlington, C.L. and Smith, P.F. "Impairment and recovery on a food foraging task following unilateral vestibular deafferentation in rats." *Hippocampus, 16*(4):368-378, 2006.

Zheng, Y., Darlington, C.L. and Smith, P.F. "Bilateral labyrinthectomy causes long-term deficit in object recognition in rat." *Neuroreport, 15*(12):1913-1916, 2004.

CHAPTER TEN
PRESSURE

Although encased in solid bone, the inner ear is not sealed off from pressure changes occurring either inside or outside the body. A normal ear isn't bothered by the pressure changes of everyday life but some Ménière's ears are.

There is a connection between the fluid spaces of the inner ear and those of the brain. Increases in the fluid pressure of the brain are passed into the inner ear, particularly in people under age 70. This has no affect on a normal inner ear. Increased blood pressure, coughing, sneezing, vomiting, straining on the toilet, lifting weights, holding breath, holding the head below the level of the heart, and being hit on the head can all increase the brain fluid pressure and therefore the inner ear pressure causing symptoms in susceptible ears.

We are all surrounded by atmospheric pressure here on earth. This pressure travels to the outer surface of the eardrum through the ear canal. It travels to the inner surface of the eardrum through the eustachian tube as well. The pressure must be the same on both sides of the eardrum for the drum to move normally when hit by sound waves.

Normal eardrum movement is not a problem for the normal ear but can be a problem for some Ménière's ears. The saccule of the inner ear can become very swollen in Ménière's. When abnormally large the saccule can apparently be stimulated by inward movement of the oval window. Whenever the eardrum moves inward from sound waves or increased atmospheric pressure the saccule is pushed and can cause symptoms. Decreases in pressure due to weather changes, mountain travel and flying have also been reported to produce symptoms in some people with Ménière's.

Increased pressure → Eardrum → malleus → incus → stapes → oval window → saccule

If the eustachian tube is too wide the eardrum may move further than normal causing symptoms in the Ménière's ear. When the tube is too narrow pressure cannot equalize, inside pressure cannot equal the outside pressure.

Malfunction of the eustachian tube has also been implicated by physicians in Europe as causing or aggravating symptoms in the Ménière's ear. These physicians advocate insertion of a ventilation tube. This tube allows pressure directly into the middle ear through the eardrum thereby equalizing pressure on both sides of the eardrum.

Pressure changes are not completely bad news for the Ménière's ear. Manipulation of pressure is also the basis for pressure treatments with the Meniett, based on research from Sweden.

SPECIAL PRESSURE SITUATIONS:
Flying:
Although modern commercial airliners are pressurized it isn't to sea level, it's to the equivalent of 6,000-8,000 feet of elevation. When taking off from Colorado Springs, Colorado cabin pressure changes from 0 to 2,000 feet in the first 20-30 minutes. When taking off from Boston it's a 6,000-8,000 foot change in that same 20 to 30 minutes. The amount of pressure change is determined by the elevation of the airport.

Some people experience symptoms while undergoing the pressure change of flying and others don't. There have even been scattered stories of improvement when flying.

What can help with this pressure change? Chewing gum, swallowing liquids, sucking on hard candy, use of EarPlanes®, decongestant nose spray, oral decongestant and clearing the ears can all be useful. Before using any of these last interventions have a discussion with your doctor to determine if they are right for you.

Scuba diving:
Submerging the head in water causes the greatest of all pressure effects on the ear; more than flying. The pressure at 10 feet (3 meters) below the surface is great enough to burst an eardrum. The pressure at 30 feet below the surface is twice atmospheric pressure at sea level. Scuba diving has the potential to damage even a normal ear.

If you have Ménière's disease DO NOT SCUBA DIVE until discussing it completely with an ear specialist to fully understand the risks and options. The pressure change could cause irritation of the saccule and vertigo resulting in symptoms when not even having an attack. There's also the chance of motion sickness. A Ménière's attack underwater could easily prove fatal from both vomiting and disorientation.

REFERENCES:

Ahsan, S.F., Standring, R. and Wang Y. "Systematic review and meta-analysis of Meniett therapy for Meniere's disease." *Laryngoscope, 125*(1):203-208, 2015.

Brattmo, M., Tideholm, B. and Carlborg, B. "Inadequate opening capacity of the eustachian tube in Ménière's disease." *Acta Otolaryngologica, 132*(3):255-260, 2012.

Kitahara, M., Kodama, A., Izukura, H. and Ozawa, H. "Effect of atmospheric pressure on hearing in patients with Meniere's disease." *Acta Otolaryngologica Supplement, 510*:111-112, 1994.

Park, J.J., Luecke, K., Luedeke, I., Emmerling, O. and Westhofen, M. "Long-term middle ear pressure measurements in inner ear disorders." *Acta Otolaryngologica, 132*(3):266-270, 2012.

Park, J.J., Chen, Y.S. and Westhofen, M. "Ménière's disease and middle ear pressure: vestibular function after transtympanic tube placement." *Acta Otolaryngologica, 129*(12):1408-1413, 2009.

CHAPTER ELEVEN
FEMALE HORMONE EFFECT

Is there a female hormone effect on Ménière's disease? There have been no large studies looking at female hormonal effects but a small 1992 study of 109 women found that 6 had symptom increases during their premenstrual time. There are individual case reports of changes during pregnancy as well. Other research looking at the affect of female hormones on hearing found increased hearing sensitivity around the time of ovulation. The evidence is not overwhelming but there does seem to be an effect in some women.

Women and men differ chemically. Women are more susceptible to some diseases including migraines, autoimmune diseases, orthostatic hypotension and osteoporosis. The eye pressure of glaucoma seems to increase during the premenstrual period in some women and some tumors grow faster in women. On the flip side woman have lower rates of cardiovascular disease during their childbearing years. Pregnant women have a higher incidence of tinnitus (ringing in the ears) with 25% experiencing it compared to 10% of the non-pregnant population.

MENSTRUAL CYCLE

The purpose of the menstrual cycle is to prepare the body for pregnancy through changes that will allow a fertilized egg to attach to the wall of the uterus. This happens through the use of chemicals called hormones. Estrogen is one of the prominent hormones during this time and its increase tends to cause fluid retention.

Many woman gain weight, have breast swelling/tenderness and complain about feeling bloated during the premenstrual time. A Ménière's ear isn't able to handle fluids like a normal ear and, apparently, has even more difficulties during the premenstrual time, for some woman.

The blood is also thicker and stickier during this time, which theoretically could lead to impaired inner ear circulation and potentially to symptoms.

PREGNANCY

Pregnancy is a time when a great many female hormones are made and changes in body fluids take place. There are both fluid retention and changes in circulation during this time.

No studies have looked into pregnancy and Ménière's disease although there are a few case reports:

- A woman had increased attacks during her pregnancy (1997).

- A woman had improvement during both pregnancies and increased problems during her premenstrual time.

- A woman had temporary recovery of her hearing loss (2014).

Studies of hearing in pregnant woman have found 25 to as many as 33% experience tinnitus (10% of the non-pregnant population have it) and 24% have aural fullness. Both tinnitus and aural fullness stop after the pregnancy. There are decreases in hearing as well, in some studies.

Why is this? Or, why isn't it? This is one more of those Ménière's disease mysteries. Not just why woman experience this but the flip side, why so many do not experience it.

REFERENCES:

Al-Mana, D., Ceranic, B., Djahanbakhch, O. and Luxon, L.M. "Hormones and the auditory system: a review of physiology and pathophysiology." *Neuroscience, 153:*881-900, 2008.

Al-Mana, D., Ceranic, B., Djahanbakhch, O. and Luxon, L.M. "Alteration in auditory function during the ovarian cycle." *Hearing Research, 268*(1-2):114-122, 2010.

Andrews, J.C. and Honrubia, V. "Premenstrual exacerbation of Ménière's disease revisited." *Otolaryngological Clinics of North America, 43:*1029-1040, 2010.

Andrews, J., Ator, G.A. and Honrubia, V. "The exacerbation of symptoms in Ménière's Disease during the premenstrual period." *Archives of Otolaryngology-Head and Neck Surgery, 118:*74-78, 1992.

Cox, J.R. "Hormonal influence on auditory function." *Ear and Hearing, 1:*219-222, 1980.

Dalton, K. "Influence of menstruation on glaucoma." *Journal of Ophthalmology, 52:*692-696, 1967.

Morse, G.G. and House, J.W. "Changes in Ménière's disease responses as a function of the menstrual cycle." *Nursing Research, 5:*286-292, 2001.

Price, T.M., Allen, T.C., Bowyer, D.L. and Watson, T.A. "Ablation of luteal phase symptoms of Ménière's disease with leuprolide." *Archives of Otolaryngology, 120:*209-211, 1994.

Schmidt, P.M., Flores, F.T., Rossi, A.G. and Silveira, A.F. "Hearing and vestibular complaints during pregnancy." *Brazilian Journal of Otorhinolaryngology, 76*(1):29-33, 2010.

Stachenfeld, N.S. "Sex hormone effects on body fluid regulation." *Exercise Sport Science Review, 36*(3):152-159, 2008.

Stevens, M.N. and Hullar, T.E. "Improvement in sensorineural hearing loss during pregnancy." *Annals of Otology, Rhinology and Laryngology, 123*(9):614-618, 2014.

Uchide, K., Suzuki, N., Taiguchi, T., Terada, S. and Inoue, M. "The possible effect of pregnancy on Ménière's disease." *ORL,* 59:292-295, 1997.

CHAPTER TWELVE
HEREDITY

The question is heard frequently, "Is Ménière's disease genetic? Does it run in families?" The short answer: yes, at least in a small number of cases.

There are many inherited or genetic diseases of the ear. According to the Boys Town Research Registry for Hereditary Hearing Loss two to three out of every 1,000 children born in the US are deaf or hard-of-hearing and genetics are thought to be involved 50% of the time. Neurofibromatosus Type II, a rare tumor of the vestibular nerve, is inherited. In addition there is an inherited susceptibility involved in some cases of inner ear poisoning from the aminoglycoside antibiotics.

Isolated reports of multiple family members developing Ménière's disease have been in the medical literature since 1941. There are also reports of multiple family members experiencing both hearing loss and vestibular symptoms that don't quite meet the diagnostic criteria for Ménière's disease. The idea that Ménière's disease could be genetic, at least in some cases, makes a lot of sense.

In the only study of an entire town, Swedish researchers found 91 people with Ménière's disease and of these 14% had family members with the disorder. In a Brazilian study 6 out of the 8 patients receiving the Ménière's diagnosis over a two-year period had a family member with it. Finnish researchers studied 118 people with Ménière's disease and found 15% had other family members with the disorder.

Ménière's disease was found to be autosomal dominant in these cases, if one parent has the gene for Ménière's disease each of the children have a 50% chance of developing the disorder.

A German study of 193 people with Ménière's disease found 37 had other family members with the disorder. Researchers then studied 19 families with a total of 81 members and found 52 of these also had Ménière's disease. Study of their DNA lead the researchers to conclude: "The Family trees suggest an autosomal dominant inheritance with reduced penetrance and anticipation. A probable candidate region for MD was located on chromosome 5."

Genetic research has not been limited to trying to discover the gene(s) causing Ménière's disease. Researchers from one study suggest genes may also have a role in bringing on the attacks of the disorder.

This type research is very basic and might not contribute to better diagnosis or treatment any time soon but is important to gain a better basic understanding of this mysterious disorder.

REFERENCES:

Arweiler-Harbeck, D., Horsthemke, B., Jahnke, K. and Hennies, H.C. "Genetic aspects of familial Meniere's disease." *Otology and Neurotology, 32*(4)695-700, 2011.

Birgerson, L., Gustavson, K.H. and Stahle, J. "Familial Meniere's disease: a genetic investigation." *American Journal of Otology, 8*(4):323-326, 1987.

Fransen, E., Verstreken, M., Verhagen, W.I., Wuyts, F.L., Huygen, P.L., D'Haese, P., Robertson, N.G., Morton, C.C., McGuirt, W.T., Smith, R.J., Declau, F., Van de Heyning, P.H. and Van Camp, G. "High prevalence of symptoms of Meniere's disease in three families with a mutation in the COCH gene." *Human Molecular Genetics, 8(*8):1425-1429. 1999.

Fung, K., Xie, Y., Hall, S.F., Lillicrap, D.P. and Taylor, S.A. "Genetic basis of familial Meniere's disease." *Journal of Otolaryngology, 31*(1):1-4, 2002.

Gazquez, I. and Lopez-Escamez, J.A. "Genetics of Recurrent Vertigo and Vestibular Disorders." *Current Genomics, 12*:443-450 443, 2011.

Klockars, T. and Kentala, E. "Inheritance of Meniere's disease in the Finnish population." *Archives of Otolaryngology Head and Neck Surgery, 133*(1):73-77, 2007.

Klar, J., Frykholm, C., Friberg, U. and Dahl, N.A. "Meniere's disease gene linked to chromosome 12p12.3." *American Journal of Medical Genetics. Part B, Neuropsychiatric Genetics, 141*(5):463-467, 2006.

Morrison, A.W. and Johnson, K.J. "Genetics (molecular biology) and Meniere's disease." *Otolaryngologic Clinics of North America, 35*(3):497-516, 2002.

Oliveira, C.A., Ferrari, I. and Messias, C.I. "Occurrence of familial Meniere's syndrome and migraine in Brasilia." *Annals of Otology, Rhinology and Laryngology, 111*(3 Pt 1):229-236, 2002.

Oliveira, C.A. and Braga, A.M. "Meniere's syndrome inherited as an autosomal dominant trait." *Annals of Otology, Rhinology and Laryngology, 101*(7):590-594, 1992.

Sekine, K., Morita, K., Masuda, K., Sato, G., Rokutan, K. and Takeda, N. "Microarray analysis of stress-related gene expression in patients with Ménière's disease." *ORL Journal of Otorhinolaryngology and Related Specialties, 67*(5):294-299, 2005.

Vrabec, J.T., Liu, L., Li, B. and Leal, S.M. "Sequence Variants in Host Cell Factor C1 Are Associated With Ménière's Disease." *Otology and Neurotology, 29*(4): 561–566, 2008.

SECTION III
DIAGNOSING MÉNIÈRE'S DISEASE

The diagnosis of many common problems is clear-cut because an accurate test is available. A strep throat can be diagnosed with a throat swab test, a broken arm with an x-ray, anemia with a blood test, ripped knee cartilage with an MRI, sinus problems with a CT scan, cancer with a biopsy and a heart attack with an ECG/blood test.

Ménière's disease isn't like this, it doesn't have a similar clear cut diagnostic test because there are large gaps in our knowledge of how the inner ear works, how Ménière's disease changes the ear, how to detect those changes and what causes the disorder.

The structure and function of the inner ear can't be seen in a living person with current technology (although MRI research is moving in that direction). Cutting or making a hole to look inside is not done because of the catastrophic damage to both hearing and balance that could occur.

Doctors do study the inner ears of people who had vestibular symptoms during their lives, after they die. It's then assumed changes in these ears caused their problems. Unfortunately when assumptions are the basis for medical decisions there is more room for error.

Diagnosis can also be difficult because ear, nose and throat surgeons are usually the ones to diagnose and treat inner ear balance disorders but these disorders are only a small part of their training and tiny part of their practice. Their experience in this area is seldom up to the level of an otologist/neurotologist.

Another problem is that when Ménière's disease first begins, the diagnostic symptoms may not all appear at the same time. Two small studies looking at this issue found only 25% of people ultimately diagnosed with Ménière's disease had all the symptoms at the outset. The other symptoms appeared over months to years in 75% of the people. In the beginning the symptoms of Ménière's disease have a tendency to come and go erratically.

All of this adds up to a lot of difficulty both understanding and diagnosing Ménière's. Now, as in the past, the most important tool in diagnosis is the history.

Since 1995 the American Academy of Otolaryngology-Head and

Neck surgery has suggested the diagnosis only be made if there have been two "attacks" consisting of vertigo lasting 20 minutes to 24 hours that occur spontaneously and not because a person shook their head, looked up at the top shelf, watched a moving object or any other activity. In addition to vertigo, hearing loss must occur as well as either ringing in the ear or a feeling of fullness in the ear.

This organization also suggested in the past that the diagnosis of Ménière's disease be divided into four different categories: possible, probable, definite and certain shown below.

OLD DIAGNOSTIC CATEGORIES OF MÉNIÈRE'S DISEASE

Possible Ménière's disease: Episodic vertigo of the Ménière's type without documented sensorineural hearing loss, fluctuating or fixed, with disequilibrium but without definitive episodes. After other causes have been excluded.

Probable Ménière's disease: One definitive episode of vertigo. Audiometrically documented hearing loss on at least one occasion. Tinnitus or aural fullness in the treated ear. All other causes have been excluded.

Definite Ménière's disease: Two or more definitive spontaneous episodes of vertigo 20 minutes or longer. Audiometrically documented hearing loss on at least one occasion. Tinnitus or aural fullness in the treated ear. Other causes excluded.

Certain Ménière's disease: Definite Ménière's disease, plus histopathologic confirmation (examination after death).

The new diagnostic categories are probable and definite as seen in the box below.

NEW DIAGNOSTIC CATEGORIES OF MÉNIÈRE'S DISEASE

Probable

Two or more episodes of vertigo or dizziness; each lasting 20 minutes to 24 hours.

Fluctuating aural symptoms (hearing, tinnitus, or fullness) in the affected ear.

Definite

Two or more spontaneous episodes of vertigo, each lasting 20 minutes to 12 hours.

Audiometrically documented low to midfrequency sensorineural hearing loss in one ear defining the affected ear on at least one occasion before, during or after one episode of vertigo.

Fluctuation of cymptoms (hearing, tinnitus or fullness) in the affected ear.

Not better accounted for by another vestibular diagnosis

DEFINITIONS:

Disequilibrium – Feeling of imbalance, unsteadiness, light-headedness and balance not being quite right.

Sensorineural hearing loss – Hearing loss occurring in the inner ear, the vestibulocochlear nerve or the area of the brain receiving sound signals.

Audiometrically documented – Measurement of hearing in a soundproof room by an audiologist.

Histopathologic confirmation – Study looking for physical changes after a person's death.

In 2015 a new set of guidelines was published. These guidelines are the result of years of committee meetings by several organizations around the world including the Equilibrium Committee of the AAO-HNS, Classification Committee of the Bárány Society, the Japan Society for Equilibrium Research, the European Academy of Otology and Neurotology, and the Korean Balance Society.

The new guidelines have two criteria, definite Ménière's disease and probable Ménière's disease.

WARNING:

Some tests used during the diagnosis of Ménière's disease are very expensive. Every insurance company has it's own policies regarding which tests are medically necessary and proven to be of clinical value. Not all tests are covered by all insurance companies.

Although doctors offices and test facilities are well versed in insurance coverage they don't always know everything about the 100's of medical insurances their patients use. Before going for testing it's important to read your insurance documents, research their web site and check with the company directly if there is any doubt about specific test coverage. When it comes to payment the policyholder has the final responsibility, be careful.

REFERENCES:

"Committee on Hearing and Equilibrium Guidelines for the Diagnosis and Evaluation of Therapy in Ménière's Disease." *Otolaryngology-Head and Neck Surgery, 113*(3): 181-185, 1995.

Goebel, J. "2015 Equilibrium Committee Amendment to the 1995 AAO-HNS Guidelines for the Definition of Ménière's Disease." *Otolaryngology-Head and Neck Surgery,* 154(3):403-404, 2016.

Lopez-Escamez, J.A., Carey, J., Chung, W.H., Goebel, J.A., Magnusson, M., Mandalà, M., Newman-Toker, D.E., Strupp, M., Suzuki, M., Trabalzini, F. and Bisdorff, A. "Diagnostic criteria for Menière's disease. Consensus document of the Bárány Society, the Japan Society for Equilibrium Research, the European Academy of Otology and Neurotology (EAONO), the American Academy of Otolaryngology-Head and Neck Surgery (AAO-HNS) and the Korean Balance Society." *Journal of Vestibular Research, 25*:1-5, 2015.

Syed, I. and Aldren, C. "Meniere's disease: an evidence based approach to assessment and management." *International Journal of Clinical Practice, 66*:166–170, 2012.

CHAPTER THIRTEEN
WHICH DOCTOR

"Whom should I go to for my Ménière's disease?" Great question—complicated answer. Some people with Ménière's disease don't require much from their health care providers while others do. Finding the right doctor can be difficult and in the end require some luck, but knowing a bit about the system can help.

A primary care provider (PCP) or general practitioner (GP) is the first stop. A GP is generally a medical or osteopathic doctor. PCP's can be a medical doctor (MD), osteopathic doctor (OD), adult or family nurse practitioner (ANP or FNP) or physician's assistant (PA). (In some insurance schemes they are also called gatekeepers because they must be consulted for all aspects of a person's medical care). This health care professional sees a person as someone with a mind, soul and a complete set of interacting body parts. They can check to see where they think symptoms are coming from and make a specialist referral if they suspect Ménière's disease or don't know what's wrong.

A primary care provider is more or less responsible for the entire body. For more complicated problems the body is divided up amongst the various specialists. In the U.S. the ear falls within the area of otolaryngology-head and neck surgery.

THE SPECIALISTS

Otolaryngologists (ENT'S)

Otolaryngologists, many times referred to as ENT's (ear, nose and throat), since it's much easier to say, deal with everything above the shoulders except the brain, mind, eyes and teeth. This is a huge amount of territory with many disorders. Cancer of the mouth, tongue, throat and voice box; plastic surgery for cleft lip and palate; nosebleeds and broken noses; tonsils, sinuses, sometimes allergy work, facial bone fractures, thyroid removal, broken jaws, salivary gland problems, external ear infections, difficulty swallowing, taste disturbances, difficulty with speech, some esophagus problems, middle ear infections, eustachian tube dysfunction, ear balance and hearing problems, and even more, are all included in this specialty.

The first step in becoming an otolaryngologist, after medical school, is a one-year internship throughout a hospital followed by a one-year general surgical residency. Then there are four years of otolaryngology residency, regulated by the American Board of Medical Specialties, ABMS. This is really an on-the-job training course or apprenticeship for doctors. A resident is on duty and on-call long hours each week and learns by working under other residents a year or two their senior and under experienced doctors who have previously completed a residency program.

Doctors become board certified in otolaryngology-head and neck surgery after completing this long residency program and successfully passing both written and oral tests. Once successful they can place the initials FACS after their name (Fellow in the American College of Surgery) and be referred to as a Diplomate of the American College of Surgery.

Most of their training time is spent hunched over the operating table learning and practicing all the skills needed to be a competent surgeon. The remaining time is used to learn about the diagnosis and non-surgical treatment of all the ear, nose, throat, head and neck disorders.

Despite all this, some otolaryngologists do good work with inner ear balance disorders. Others just don't have the education or experience to be effective, particularly in complicated cases or when symptoms don't fit the "textbook" description.

Otology and Neurotology

 Because the structure and function of the inner ear are so specialized and complicated there are sub-specialties within otolaryngology-head and neck surgery focusing just on the ear and the inner ear. One small study has found that "Neurotologists tend to use a wider variety of medications in their treatment protocols than generalists."

The two ear sub-specialties are, otology and neurotology. Otology covers all aspects of the ear and neurotology covers the inner ear and its role in balance and hearing. Although in theory these are different areas of expertise, in practice most ear doctors are both otologists and neurotologists.

Many doctors using the title have undergone further training, beyond their residency, called a fellowship. A fellowship is another formal on-the-job program that takes place after the residency and board certification are completed. During fellowship training a physician spends their time learning about the ear and it's disorders along with diagnosis and treatment. This training lasts one to two years and again generally includes a lot of time learning surgery. Different fellowship programs have different focuses with some preparing doctors to do scientific research or teach in a university and others focusing more on skills for private practice.

These fellowships were not standardized nor was certification testing offered until the American Board of Otolaryngology (www.aboto.org) began offering it in 2004.

Not everyone who has successfully completed a fellowship in otology or neurotology limits his or her practice to these areas. Many continue to practice in other areas of the otololaryngology-head and neck specialty. Otolaryngology-head and neck surgery is a specialty, doctors practicing it are specialists and anything within their specialty is what they specialize in. If you ask, "Do you specialize in inner ear balance disorders?" the answer of yes from anyone board certified as an otolaryngologist is honest even if it is only one of many areas they practice in.

To make sure a doctor solely practices on folks with ear disorders ask if they limit their practice to ear disorders, not if they specialize in them.

Neurologists
Neurologists are medical doctors specializing in the medical treatment of disorders of the nervous system (brain, spinal cord and nerves) and muscles. According to the American Board of Psychiatry and Neurology these disorders include stroke, brain and spinal cord tumors, muscular dystrophy, headache and other pain, meningitis, encephalitis, epilepsy and seizures, Parkinson's disease, Alzheimer's, multiple sclerosis and the effects of systemic disease on the nervous system. They usually don't have special training in ear disease or disorders of hearing.

A board certified neurologist has completed four years of post medical school residency training with at least three years in neurology and successfully completed a rigorous certification process. Unlike their otolaryngologist colleagues none of this time is spent in the operating room.

Some have had fellowship training in neurotology or what is sometimes referred to as otoneurology and limit their practice to people with vestibular problems

SELECTING A SPECIALIST
There's a lot to consider when selecting a specialist. Will insurance pay or decide? Will you try to find a specialist on your own or use your PCP? Which type of specialist? What's available? Some entire states

have no practicing neurotologist or otoneurologist. The easiest thing to do is have a primary care provider decide on the specialist. Relying on their experience will lift a large burden. However, this sounds easier than it usually is. Balance disorders are such a specialized little area of medicine some primary care providers don't know enough about them to select the best specialist. An MD's basic education doesn't include much about the inner ear. Most medical schools only require an hour or two of general lectures about the inner ear in their entire 4-year curriculum. A UK study found GP's usually didn't have detailed knowledge about Ménière's disease and some weren't even aware of the National Health Service guidelines for the disorder.

Another problem is that most GP's and PCP's will refer their patients to other doctors in their group or medical building or their hospital, not necessarily to the best specialist available in the area. Want to see the very best? Insist. Ask them whom they would send their spouse, mother, or children to.

An HMO (Health Maintenance Organization) or PPO (Preferred provider organization) will first send a subscriber to one of their primary care providers. Then, if they determine a specialist is needed it will be with whomever they have a contract. Sometimes this happens to be the best person in the area; other times it's someone without special training or experience in inner ear balance disorders who might even dislike seeing "dizzy" people.

If this happens to you complain in writing and by telephone. Tell the insurance people who the proper specialist is. Not good at insisting? Don't be bashful; enlist the help of a relative or friend who is good at it.

Don't want to leave finding a specialist in the hands of someone else? That's OK but this will mean more work and soul searching for you.

The yellow pages list otolaryngologists and otologists in their "Physician's and Surgeon's" listings. A listing may include if the doctor limits their practice in any way. To find out if they are board certified or have done an otology/neurotology fellowship call their office and ask or check in "The Official ABMS Directory of Board Certified Medical Specialists" at the local library, on the Internet at www.abms.org or via toll free number, 1-866-275-2267. Otolaryngolgists can be located through the American Academy of Otolaryngology-Head and Neck Surgery webpage, www.entnet.org/ent_otolaryngologist.cfm Both the American Neurotology Society and the American Otological Society have membership lists on their WebPages:

www.americanneurotologysociety.com/membership.html
www.americanotologicalsociety.org/membership.html

Other people with Ménière's disease can be found on the Internet or through patient organizations like the Vestibular Disorders Association (VEDA) in the U.S. VEDA's addresses are www.vestibular.org and P.O. Box 4467, Portland, OR, 92708–4467. In Canada there is the Balance and Dizziness Disorders Society of Vancouver, B.C., www.balanceanddizziness.org, 325 - 5525 West Blvd., Vancouver, B.C. V6M 3W6, (604) 878-8383.

There are English-speaking organizations outside of North America.

- UK: The Ménière's Society at http://www.menieres.org.uk/ and The Rookery, Surrey Hills Business Park, Wotton, Dorking, Surrey, RH5 6QT, 0845 120 2975.

- Australia: Ménière's Australia www.menieres.org.au

Don't want to go to a surgeon? It's a lot harder to find a neurologist with training in neurotology. UCLA, Johns Hopkins, the Cleveland Clinic, Emory University, Wake Forest University, Massachusetts Eye and Ear Infirmary and the University of Pittsburgh are some institutions where they can be found.

PhD VERSUS MD

During diagnosis or treatment you may run into a health car professional with a PhD. How does a Ph.D. differ from an M.D.? An M.D. is a physician, someone who practices medicine including making medical diagnoses and treating disease one person at a time. A Ph.D. is a scientist trained in performing scientific research in one area of science with groups of people or lab animals. They differ not only in what they do but also in the education they have.

The educational path for an M.D. in the U.S. is 4 years in college studying a subject such as zoology, biology, electrical engineering or a host of other things to earn a bachelor's degree. They then go on to medical school that is generally 4 years in length with the first two years spent studying science and the last two learning and doing the practice of medicine. After passing a rigorous examination they receive their MD from the state licensing board and in theory can go off and independently practice medicine.

In reality nearly every medical school graduate goes into residency training programs that are paid, on the job learning experiences lasting three of more years depending upon the type medicine they are studying. Surgeons spend the most time in residencies because learning and practicing surgery requires more time.

Getting an MD does not require a master's degree and usually does not focus on scientific research nor does it usually require completion of a large research project to graduate.

The PhD's education begins with an undergraduate degree in their area of interest such as audiology, psychology or biology. Two more years are spent earning a master's degree in their chosen field of science followed by four or more years earning a PhD. The PhD years revolve around a very large research study designed and carried out by the student. A document, typically hundreds of pages long, called a dissertation, is written describing the research. A committee of professors must find the dissertation acceptable during a rigorous question and answer period. This schoolwork is followed by a year or two working as a "post-doc" doing research while loosely supervised by another more experienced PhD.

Scientific research is an integral part of attaining a PhD. The process is studied for years and the student designs and carries out their own research in order to complete their degrees.

Some doctors have the title, M.D./PhD. Some medical school programs automatically bestow this double degree without extra work from the student while others require more work and/or time to earn it. An M.D./PhD is seldom someone who has earned both degrees separately.

REFERENCES:

American board of Psychiatry and Neurology, http://www.abpn.com, accessed August, 4, 2015.

American Neurotology Society, http://www.americanneurotologysociety.com, accessed May, 2017.

American Otological Society, http://www.americanotological.org, accessed May, 2017.

_____. *The Official ABMS Directory of Board Certified Medical Specialists*, Vol. 3, Otolaryngologists, 32 edition. Saunders, 2010.

Clyde, J.W., Oberman, B.S. and Isildak, H. "Current management practices in Meniere's Disease." *Otology and Neurotology*, 38(6):159-167, 2017.

Smale, E., McDonald, S., Maha, N. and Short, S. "Management of Ménière's disease in general practice: adherence to the UK National Health Service 'Prodigy' guidelines." *Journal of Laryngology and Otology*, 27:1-6, 2007.

CHAPTER FOURTEEN
SPECIALIST VISIT

What will the trip to a specialist be like? An initial visit to the specialist usually has two parts: the history and the examination. In some practices a hearing test will be done before seeing the doctor; in others it's done at another time and/or location.

Wear something comfortable for this appointment and take someone along who can help you get home – on occasion it can bring on a temporary increase in symptoms or the temporary appearance of new ones.

HISTORY

The most crucial step in figuring out what's wrong and determining a treatment is hearing the full story. What's being experienced now? When did it start? What makes it worse? Does anything help it? Without this sort of information even $10,000 worth of tests most likely won't produce an accurate diagnosis.

Listening to a history isn't polite; it's crucial for an appropriate diagnosis. Without this information they can't formulate a working diagnosis, determine the appropriate tests needed or design a personalized treatment plan. If the doctor you see won't listen to your story don't waste time with them, get yourself someone who will listen.

Keep a diary of your activities, what you eat, where you go and how you feel, what you are experiencing. If you have trouble thinking and speaking in an organized fashion it might be a good idea to get your story or history organized before seeing a doctor for the first time. When you're prepared there's less chance of leaving something out or giving a confused story a doctor might not be able to follow.

Doctor's are only human and may not be able to stay completely attentive during long explanations and stories. Try to keep to the facts, if feeling lightheaded say so plainly and clearly, don't launch into your theories of where it's coming from unless asked. Keep it short, sweet and accurate; don't leave anything out but stay on topic and don't meander.

Stay away from one-word descriptions like "vertigo." If having episodes of spinning say that, don't call it vertigo. Be sure your doctor knows exactly what you mean because their definition of vertigo, and other words, may differ from yours. Don't ever assume your definition is the same as theirs.

Should you walk into an appointment with a printed history and diary? Good question. Some doctors have a questionnaire for you to fill out, so writing something ahead of time could be a waste of time and effort. If they don't have a questionnaire, your own written summary would be helpful. On the other hand a doctor could feel intimidated by your preparation or feel your real problem is being wrapped up in concerns about your body.

What they'll want to know about your symptoms
- What are your symptoms?
- When did they begin?
- Have they occurred before?
- What was happening when first experienced?
- Are they always the same or do they increase or decrease?
- What causes them to increase or decrease?
- Does anything stop them?
- Do they come in episodes?
- How severe are they?
- Do the symptoms stay the same? Increase or decrease?
- Any drugs being taken or special diet eaten?
- The general health of blood relatives.
- Are nausea and vomiting present?
- Is there tinnitus or a hearing loss?
- Sensitive to sounds of any sort?
- Does anything seem to bring them on?
- Any ear infections in the past?
- Do relatives have similar symptoms now, or in the past?
- Any allergies or hay fever now or in the past?
- Ever had migraines?

Giving your doctor an accurate and thorough history is the first and most important step on the way to a diagnosis. It's every bit as important as an examination or any test.

The next step after giving a history is an examination. This, coupled with the history, may provide enough information to make a diagnosis. If not, the examination should help determine what tests would be useful.

EXAMINATION

What the examination consists of has a lot to do with the type specialist you see. An otolaryngologist may begin with a general ear, nose and throat exam including looking in the nose and at the vocal cords in addition to looking in the ears. An otologist or neurologist may stay entirely focused on the ear checking hearing, the external ear and balance function. A neurologist specializing in dizziness might spend more time looking at the function of the neurological system.

A thorough exam by any of these specialists should include checks of the:

- Ear

- Hearing

- Brain and nervous system (selected areas)

- Balance and body movement

- Eye movement

The external ear canal can be checked for infection, wax buildup, the presence of a foreign body as well as holes in the eardrum. They can also check for middle ear fluid, infection and an ear growth called a cholesteatoma. Hearing should be tested in a sound proof booth by an audiologist.

Because some brain and nervous system diseases can cause symptoms similar to those of Ménière's disease, a very limited neurological examination is done. Eye movement, pupil reaction to light, the inside of the eyes, the ability to touch the nose with an index finger, facial muscle movement, movement coordination, how a person walks, how their senses are functioning and the ability to answer questions are all checked.

Several tests of balance consisting of variations in standing and walking can be done during an office exam.

- One of the oldest tests in use is the Romberg. It is done standing quietly with arms at the sides (or possibly held straight out in front) and feet side by side with eyes open and then closed. The doctor stands close by to steady someone in the unlikely event they start to fall. A more modern addition to the test may also be done by standing with one foot in front of the other, toes of one foot touching the heel of the other, with arms folded across the chest, eyes open and then eyes closed.

- Routine walking with eyes open and then closed and walking heel to toe, one foot in front of the other with the eyes open and possibly with them closed.

- Fukoda stepping test: marching in place with the eyes closed and arms held straight out in front. You might be asked to hold a smartphone (with a special app.) while doing this test.

The eyes will be observed for nystagmus (eye jerking) while staring at the finger of the examiner or at a light and may also be observed while moving the head. In addition they may look for nystagmus while moving the head back and forth or when the examiner moves it. They may also watch while you cough or strain. You may be asked to tilt the head forward and then shake the head back and forth for 30 seconds. They may examine your eyes while moving you from a sitting to laying position, a test called the Dix-Hallpike. They might move your head and ask you to read a Snellen chart (eye testing chart).

After the history and examination, including hearing test, the specialist should have enough information to make a diagnosis, prescribe a treatment, determine what tests should be done or all of these.

REFERENCES:

Baloh, R.W. and Honrubia, V. *Clinical neurophysiology of the vestibular system.* Fourth edition. Oxford: Oxford University Press, 2010.

Brandt, T. and Strupp, M. "General vestibular testing." *Clinical Neurophysiology, 116*:406–426, 2005.

Goebel, J.A. *Practical Management of the Dizzy Patient* Philadelphia: Lippincott Williams and Wilkins 2nd ed, 2008.

Jacobson, G. and Shepard, N. *Balance Function Assessment and Management.* San Diego: Plural Publishing, 2nd ed, 2015.

Kheradmand, A. and Zee, D.S. "The bedside examination of the vestibulo-ocular reflex (VOR): an update." *Reviews of Neurology (Paris), 168*(10):710-719, 2012.

McNaboe, E. and Kerr, A. "Why history is the key in the diagnosis of vertigo." *Practitioner, 244*(1612):648-653, 2000.

Rosenberg, M.L. and Gizzi, M. "Neuro-otologic history." *Otolaryngologic Clinics of North America, 33(3):471-482, 2000.*

Whittaker, M., Mathew, A., Kanani, R. and Kanegaonkar, R.G. "Assessing the Unterberger test: introduction of a novel smartphone application." *Journal of Laryngology and Otology, 128*(11):958-960, 2014.

Zamysłowska-Szmytke, E., Szostek-Rogula, S. and Śliwińska-Kowalska, M. "Bedside examination for vestibular screening in occupational medicine." *International Journal of Occupational, Medical and Environmental Health, 28*(2):379-387, 2015.

CHAPTER FIFTEEN
VESTIBULAR TESTS

Current tests of vestibular function aren't as good as we'd like because the interior of the inner ear can't be seen and the vestibular information going to the brain via the vestibulo-cochlear nerve can't be directly measured. Tests can help evaluate three of the vestibular reflexes, the vestibulo-ocular reflex (VOR), the vestibulo-spinal reflex (VSR) and the vestibullo-collic reflex (VCR). Sadly many tests can only determine if there is a problem, not which problem. Some can't even determine which ear has the problem.

Testing tries to answer four basic questions:
- Is the problem in the inner ear?
- Which ear?
- Which disease?
- How bad is the disease?

Tests are used in Ménière's disease to determine if vestibular function has been reduced or lost, to rule out some other conditions that could cause the symptoms and evaluate balance ability/disability over time. The tests include electronystagmography (ENG), rotational tests, computerized dynamic posturography, dynamic visual acuity and vestibular evoked myogenic potential (VEMP).

TEST PREPARATION
Complete preparation instructions should be provided by the staff of the doctor's office or the testing center. These will include when to show up, how much time to allow for the testing, how to prepare and what drugs should be stopped before testing. In general, anti-vertigo drugs like meclizine (Antivert, Dramamine Less Drowsy) and dimenhydrinate (Dramamine Original), antivomiting drugs like Phenergan and Compazine, painkillers, sleep aids and alcohol are stopped 24 to 48 hours before the test. Any questions about drugs should be addressed to the doctor's office or the test facility staff.

People with neck or back problems, a false eye, or strabismus, contact lenses or vision so poor they can't see without glasses should inform the doctors' office and the testing center before making an appointment.

Wear comfortable clothing for these tests. Don't wear a dress or skirt, and don't use make-up on the day of testing because many of these tests include placing sticky patches on the face. Arrange to be driven home since the tests occasionally stir up symptoms and fatigue.

ELECTRONYSTAGMOGRAPHY
(ENG)/VIDEONYSTAGMOGRAPHY (VNG)
Probably the most widely used vestibular testing. Both look at the vestibulo-ocular reflex (the reflex using vestibuar information to move the eyes) and is Although called electronystagmography, the ENG can measure more than just nystagmus and can also record eye movements having nothing to do with the inner ear. The results can help determine if the brain is the cause of symptoms, particularly the cerebellum, instead of the inner ear.

It's an ENG when electrodes are used for measurement and a VNG when using videonystragmography (uses eye goggles instead of electrodes).

Nystagmus is a jerking of the eyes that can be horizontal (back and forth), vertical (up and down), or rotary (circular). It has two parts or phases, a slow and a fast. The slow phase is created by the vestibular system and the fast phase by the brain. The eyes slowly move toward one inner ear and the brain snaps the eyes back to center once their movement is detected.

An ENG/VNG is really several tests including:
- Visual tracking (can also be called visual-ocular control, ocular dysmetria testing)
- Optokinetic nystagmus
- Optokinetic after-nystagmus
- Saccades testing or saccadic tracking
- Smooth pursuit or sinusoidal tracking
- Spontaneous nystagmus
- Gaze
- Positional testing
- Positioning (Hallpike) testing
- Fistula or pressure testing
- Head shaking
- Caloric (may also be called bithermal caloric, monothermal caloric)

The initials "ENG" or "VNG" most likely will not be on a bill or statement. A list of the various tests will appear on the bill.

The test and its preparation generally require at least 60 minutes. First, areas around the eyes are cleaned and electrodes applied so eye movements can be electrically monitored during the test. Because blinking interferes with interpretation, do not blink during the test. Also, no gum chewing during testing.

When tested with goggles, the eyes are kept open all of the time. The goggles look a bit like ski goggles, are more comfortable than electrodes and can pick up any eye movement, including rotary and vertical, not just horizontal.

During this testing many instructions are given such as follow this or that with your eyes, stare at this or that, stare at something moving, stare at something stationary, follow a target with only your eyes, move your eyes from here to there, close your eyes, open your eyes, turn your head, roll on your side, or count backwards from 100 by threes or name names starting with the letter A, letter B, etc.

Different positions will be used including sitting up, lying down on one side or another or turning the head to one side or another. Most of these position changes are slow except for the "Hallpike" or positioning test. In this test, position is changed rapidly from sitting to lying with the head to one side and lower than the body (called the head-hanging position) followed by a rapid return to a sitting position. After a rest, the procedure is repeated on the opposite side.

During the fistula or pressure test an earplug is placed in one ear canal, positive and then negative pressure introduced and eye movement measured. Then the other ear is tested.

The caloric test is generally done last. The majority of people having an ENG find this test to be the most uncomfortable and memorable because it can cause temporary vertigo and nausea. The most commonly administered version is the four part caloric test also called the bithermal alternating caloric. The temperature in the ear canal of each ear is temporarily changed by a few degrees a total of four times (first ear warm, second ear warm, first ear cool, second ear cool). A catheter is painlessly slid into the ear canal and air or water delivered causing a temperature change. Eye reaction is measured while performing a mental task such as counting backwards from 100 by subtracting threes or naming things starting with a certain letter. Some test centers change the temperature in both ears simultaneously instead of the more standard alternation method, and others change the temperature only once rather than twice.

The temperature change causes a spinning sensation for a short time. The most intense spinning occurs about 60 seconds into the change. The strength of the spinning depends upon the amount of vestibular function. present. Nystagmus and vertigo are expected during this temperature change, in a functioning ear. If they don't occur, the test is considered abnormal. Staring at a light or dot on the ceiling when instructed to, will usually stop the nystagmus and vertigo. (This is a tactic used by many people to lessen their vertigo during an attack of Ménière's disease).

Some people with Ménière's disease find the spinning caused by the caloric test to be similar to the spinning they experience during attacks, while others don't.

The amount and direction of the nystagmus is used to help determine if the problem is in the brain or in the inner ear and, most important, which ear is the "problem" ear.

An ENG alone can't diagnose Ménière's disease because it causes no specific change. A normal ENG does not rule it out either. A reduced response to the caloric test indicates a problem, not which one, or, where. It cannot even determine if the cause of the reduced response is located solely within the inner ear rather then in the vestibulocochlear nerve or the brain. The side of the damage and an estimate of the percentage of loss may be determined.

This test should not cause an attack of Ménière's disease (vertigo with hearing loss and increased tinnitus, or aural pressure) but can cause nausea, fatigue, and a temporary off-balance sensation. Plan to be driven home from the test, or allow enough time to recover before driving.

ROTARY CHAIR
One property of the vestibulo-ocular reflex (VOR) is that when vision is absent (in darkness or with the eyes closed), turning the head in one-direction results in movement of the eyes at exactly the same time and rate of speed in the opposite direction. The rotary chair test is designed to examine this property. The rotary chair is a computerized, passive, objective test of the horizontal vestibulo-ocular reflex (VOR). It may also be called SHAT or SHA for "sinusoidal harmonic acceleration test" or total body rotational testing.

The test is done in a small room while seated on a motor-driven computerized chair with head bent forward a bit and the lights turned off. Before beginning the test, the tester applies infrared goggles or cleans some of the face, applies electrodes to the clean areas, and puts headphones on the head for constant contact. The test and its preparation generally require 40 to 45 minutes.

The test itself has two general parts, chair movement and visual testing. In most test facilities the chair moves slowly back and forth through 180 degrees, it does not spin rapidly or round and round. During chair movement the audiologist will make requests at times such as look at this light or name ladies names starting with the letter A. Instructions will be given during the visual gaze section to find and follow a little red light with the eyes. Some testing facilities also add another part, the optokinetic drum test, with the room lights on.

The rotary chair test shows how well the VOR is working, as well as how the brain processes vestibular information and integrates visual and vestibular information.

The test can, at times, show the presence of a vestibular problem but does not usually help identify which ear has the problem. No rotary chair result by itself specifically identifies or rules out Ménière's disease. It can be used to assess how the brain is "compensating" for a permanent loss of vestibular function and can be used over time to look at this phenomenon. It's also a good test for assessing people with bilateral losses.

This test should not have any long-term effect on vestibular symptoms. Anyone who has their symptoms aggravated by movement should plan to be driven home after the test. Many people find the rotary chair test easier and more comfortable than caloric testing.

HEAD-SHAKING TEST (HSVOR)
The head-shaking test, also called the head-shaking vestibulo-ocular reflex test or HSVOR, is usually a non-computerized, passive test. The HSVOR is done sitting, usually while wearing Frenzel lenses (glasses or goggles with thick lenses that prevent focusing the eyes). The doctor or audiologist moves the head back and forth with his or her hands and observes the eyes for nystagmus.

This test produces nystagmus, the speed and direction of which are observed and sometimes recorded. An abnormal test can suggest a problem with the vestibulo-ocular reflex, either in the inner ear, the vestibular nerve, or the brain. No HSVOR result establishes the presence of Ménière's disease or, on the other hand, rules it out.

Although it can cause temporary fatigue and a feeling of imbalance, this test should not have any long-term affect on symptoms. Anyone who has their symptoms aggravated by head movement should plan to be driven home after the test.

AUTO-ROTATIONAL TESTING

A third type of rotational test, the auto-rotational test, is a computerized test objectively measuring the ability to focus on a stationary target during active head movement, both back and forth and up and down. The test is also referred to as a head-on-body rotation test, a head-only auto-rotational test, an active head rotation test, a vestibular auto-rotation test (VAT), or a vestibular-ocular reflex testing equipment test (VORTEQ). It can test the VOR both horizontally and vertically and tests the VOR at higher speeds than the rotary chair.

Electrodes are placed on the face to measure eye movement (or goggles are worn), and a device resembling a headband is placed around the head to measure the speed of head movement. While in a sitting position, you are asked to move your head back and forth in time with a sound while looking at a visual target (usually a dot) close by. The movement will be no longer than 18 seconds. This visual target may appear to jump during the test, but it actually remains stationary. The procedure is repeated twice more at different speeds and then, after a short pause up-and-down movements are done. This test requires about 20 minutes including preparation time.

An abnormal test result shows a problem with the vestibulo-ocular reflex. One published study suggests that people with Ménière's disease have a specific test result, but auto-rotation testing is not generally used alone to diagnose the disorder.

Some people have their symptoms temporarily stirred up by this test. Plan to be driven home.

COMPUTERIZED DYNAMIC POSTUROGRAPHY (CDP)

This is a computerized group of tests measuring the vestibulo-spinal reflex. Computerized dynamic posturography (CDP) can also be called dynamic posturography, moving platform p osturography, dynamic computerized platform posturography, or platform posturography.

Because the testing equipment includes a harness to prevent falling, shorts or slacks should be worn. Your shoes, and possibly socks, will be removed before starting the test.

A harness similar to those used by parachutists is worn during the test to prevent falling if a loss of balance occurs. The only requirement during the test is to stand still with hands at the sides and follow all the directions given such as eyes open, eyes closed. Instructions about when to open and close the eyes will be given.

Sometimes a pressure test will be included in CDP testing. This involves painless insertion of an earpiece into your ear canal, introducing positive and negative pressure, and measuring movement or sway. This procedure is repeated with positive and negative pressure in each ear, one ear at a time.

CDP testing shows how well balance is maintained in response to various situations, such as when information is available from vision, proprioception, and the vestibular areas vs. when information is available from only one or two of these systems or when the information is inaccurate.

Testing also measures muscle response to changing balance situations. Certain muscle "strategies" are used subconsciously and automatically to maintain balance, and these can also be assessed. Finally, CDP can measure balance response to increased and decreased pressure in each ear.

CDP may only indicate if a problem is present and not if the trouble is in the inner ear, nerve, or brain. A possible exception is pressure testing done one ear at a time. There is no specific CDP result found in Ménière's disease.

Because this test shows muscle responses, some doctors use it not only to make a diagnosis but, to determine if some type of physical therapy might help. The test can also be repeated from time to time to document changes in balance ability.

This testing can cause momentary spatial disorientation, confusion about position in space, and possibly some fatigue, plan to be driven home.

DYNAMIC VISUAL ACUITY TEST

Dynamic visual acuity testing is done to check on vision during head movement. It can be done by simply trying to read a vision or Snellen chart while moving the head back and forth or up and down or might be done as a computerized test.

The computerized version is done with a headband sensor in place while looking at a computer screen and moving the head in time with a computer generated beeping sound. While moving the head the testee is asked to report which way the open side of a square is facing.

There is no finding specific to Ménière's disease but vision will not be as accurate in a person with a damaged VOR as it is in someone with a normal VOR.

This test can stir up symptoms in people sensitive to head movement. Plan to be driven home afterward.

VESTIBULAR EVOKED MYOGENIC POTENTIAL (VEMP)

VEMP tests the vestibulocervical reflex (VCR), the reflex using information from the saccule of the vestibule. This original type of the test is also referred to as the cVEMP

A hearing test is done first because VEMP testing uses sound. Electrodes are then attached to the neck, breastbone and forehead. The test can be done while either lying down or sitting. In the version done lying down the head is held up off the table at times. While in the sitting version the head is turned so the chin is over the shoulder away from the side being tested while tightening or contracting the muscles. In both versions clicks and/or tone bursts are heard. No response to the sounds is required.

In someone younger than 70 years this test can show if there are problems in the saccule, brain and/or sternocleidomastoid neck muscles. Someone with Ménière's disease may have a low-amplitude or absent response but a normal test does not rule out the disorder. The test can be used over time to document the progression of Ménière's disease. Some of the disorders it can help uncover in addition to Ménière's disease are the Tullo phenomenon, perilymph fistula, superior canal dehiscence, and multiple sclerosis.

Effects from this test include muscle fatigue, increased tinnitus and dizziness in people whose symptoms are increased by loud sound.

This test continues to evolve. One area under research is the use of glycerol during the test to help diagnose Ménière's disease. Glycerol is a strong diuretic given to reduce fluid pressure in the inner ear. The test is done before drinking the bad tasting, flavored substance. The test is repeated later once the glycerol has had time to work. If the test result changes significantly it's assumed that the glycerol reduced the amount of endolymph and that Ménière's disease must be present.

Another variant being studied is the Ocular VEMP or oVEMP. It is hoped this addition to the test can look a bit more at the utricle, the other little organ inside the vestibule of the inner ear.

REFERENCES:

Adams, M.E., Heidenreich, K.D. and Kileny, P.R. "Audiovestibular testing in patients with Meniere's disease." *Otolaryngological Clinics of North America*, *43*:995-1009, 2010.

Baloh, R.W. and Honrubia, V. *Clinical neurophysiology of the vestibular system.* 4th edition. Oxford: Oxford University Press, 2010.

Brandt, T. and Strupp, M. "General vestibular testing." *Clinical Neurophysiology, 116*:406–426, 2005.

Curthoyrs, Vulvovic, V. and Manzar, L. "Ocular vestibular-evoked myogenic potential (oVEMP) to test utricular function: neural and oculomotor evidence." *Acta Otorhinolaryngologica Italica, 32*:41-45, 2012.

De Waele, C. "VEMP Induced by High Level Clicks." *Advances in Otorhinolaryngology*, *58*:98-109, 2001.

Goebel, J.A. *Practical management of the dizzy patient. 2nd edition* Philadelphia: Lippincott William & Wilkins, 2008.

Jacobson, G. and Shepard, N. *Balance Function Assessment and Management.* San Diego: Plural Publishing, 2nd ed, 2015.

Leigh, R.J. and Zee, D.S. *The Neurology of Eye Movements* 4th edition, USA: Oxford University Press, 2006.

CHAPTER SIXTEEN
HEARING TESTS

Tests of hearing are a standard part of the Ménière's workup whether or not hearing symptoms are present. Because some vestibular disorders include hearing loss and others don't, hearing tests can help rule out some diseases or make others more likely. If hearing hasn't been affected the test will serve as a baseline, to compare with future hearing tests.

An audiologist or audiology technician generally performs hearing tests. An audiologist has completed a minimum of five or six years of college studying hearing, hearing tests, and devices to aid hearing. They have earned a masters degree and passed a standardized test to become a certified audiologist with the initials CCC-A behind their name. They know more about hearing than any other licensed health care professional. An audiology technician who has less training and education may also perform the hearing tests.

People experiencing symptoms whenever they hear loud sounds or experience pressure changes should make arrangements for someone to drive them home after the testing.

PURE TONE AUDIOLOGY (PTA)

Standardized single tones at various pitches and levels of loudness are played through headphones in this test and the testee is asked to let the tester know when they are heard. Sometimes, for technical reasons, the audiologist will add a sound device behind the ear and/or the sound of static to the test. The results are charted on a graph showing the pitch/tone along one line and the decibel (loudness) level on the other.

LOUDNESS BALANCE TEST

This is a test for recruitment, abnormal loudness growth, sometimes seen in Ménière's disease. In this test the audiologist will play sounds and ask about the loudness of the sounds. If recruitment is present a sound will seem to be of the same loudness in both ears when it isn't.

SPEECH

There are two speech tests in common use, the speech reception threshold test and word recognition test. In both tests the testee is asked to repeat words spoken by the audiologist. Headphones are worn during this testing.

Speech reception threshold (SRT)

This test is designed to find out how loud words must be in order to correctly identify 50% of them. Familiar, two syllable words like cowboy and hotdog are spoken at a very quiet level, increasing in loudness until 50% of the words can be identified correctly. The test results indicate the level of loudness, also called the decibel level.

Word recognition (speech discrimination)

The aim of this test is just what the title says, word recognition. Phonetically balanced, single syllable words are spoken at 40 decibels of loudness above the speech reception threshold and the correct percentage of words identified is recorded.

IMMITTANCE AUDIOMETRY TESTS

This group of tests checks middle ear function, eardrum movement and the acoustic reflex. They are used to rule out middle ear and eustachian tube dysfunction. All are done with a soft plug in the ear canal connected to a computerized machine sending pressure or sound into the ear and measuring their effect on the ear.

Tympanogram

The testee sits quietly and does nothing during this test. Positive, then negative pressure along with sound are sent into the external ear canal. Eardrum movement is measured and printed on a graph. The shape is then interpreted to determine how well the middle ear and eustachian tube are functioning. Different conditions result in differing shapes on the graph and these shapes have letter names such as Type A and Type B.

A normal tympanogram means the eardrum is moving normally and the eustachian tube is letting atmospheric pressure into the middle ear.

Abnormalities that a tympanogram can discover include a flaccid or floppy ear drum, middle ear fluid, a scarred or thickened ear drum, perforated ear drum (hole in the ear drum) ossicular discontinuity (the little ear bones are no longer connected), glue ear, otosclerosis, and ear canal blockage.

Stapedial reflex

This test measures the acoustic reflex and is always done after the tympanogram. The acoustic reflex causes a middle ear's muscle to contract during loud sound. This muscle contraction causes the little middle ear bones to tighten up in an effort to stop all the loud sound from entering the inner ear.

In this test a sound is played through the headphones and the amount of sound coming back from the tympanic membrane measured. Some people with Ménière's disease have an odd result but this is not generally used on its own to diagnose Ménière's disease.

Having central nervous system depressants, including alcohol in the blood stream, can make the test inaccurate.

AUDITORY EVOKED RESPONSES
These tests might be used in a vestibular work-up. They measure the electrical activity created during hearing. A computer is used to send sound into the ear and interpret the electrical events from the vestibulocochlear nerve to the brain. There are two commonly used in a vestibular work-up, the ECOG and the ABR. A third, the otoacoustic emissions test, may also be used.

Auditory brainstem response (ABR)
The ABR is also called a BAER (brainstem auditory response), BSER (Brainstem evoked response) and a number of other similar things. It's done to measure the nerve activity of sound as it moves to the brain.

In this test electrodes are placed on the head and ear lobes or inserted into the ear canals, sounds are then played through headphones and the electrical waves they produce recorded with a computer.

The electrical activity is displayed as seven waves as sound moves from the ear to the brain and then within the brain. The first wave occurs in the ear and is studied in even greater detail in the next test, the electrocochleography, ECOG.

The ABR is usually done to check for the presence of an acoustic neuroma, a rare tumor of the vestibulocochlear nerve. It can also be used to show proof of a hearing loss or deafness.

Electrocochleography (ECOG)
This test is similar to the ABR (see above) but takes a closer look at the first two waves of the ABR that occur in the cochlea and along the vestibulocochlear nerve. It's thought this can show information about the hair cells of the cochlea and determine if there's an increased amount of endolymph in the inner ear. ECOG can't be done on a deaf ear.

Again, electrodes, sticky pads connected to wires, are placed on the head and ear lobes and soft tubes inserted into the ear canals, clicking sounds played through head phones and the electrical waves they produce recorded and analyzed with a computer. A ratio of the SP to AP is calculated during the test. If it's greater than normal it's thought there's too much endolymph in the inner ear.

There are usually three parts to the test, the cochlear microphonics (CM), summating potential (SP) and the action potential (AP). A bill might list these individual tests rather than the word electrocochleogram.

A 2010 study of American Otological Society and American Neurotology Society members found only 17.5% used this test routinely in the diagnosis of Ménière's disease while 46.7% did not use it all.

Otoacoustic emissions
    This test checks on the condition of hearing hair cells. Yes, the ears have actually been found to make sounds both on their own and after sound enters them.

A padded soft wire containing a microphone is painlessly inserted into the ear canal, a sound is sent into the ear, a microphone picks up any sound made by the cochlea in response and a computer then analyzes the sound.

There is no specific Ménière's disease result.

GLYCEROL TESTING
    Glycerol testing is also called a dehydration test or glycerol dehydration test. This really isn't a test but is an addition to testing. A test such as pure tone audiology, VEMP, ECOG or otoacoustic emissions is done, glycerol drunk and after a waiting period the test redone, sometimes multiple times.

Because endolymphatic hydrops is associated with Ménière's disease it's thought that a reduction in the amount of endolymph should improve test results. The glycerol testing is said to be positive if the test results improve after taking the glycerol.

The glycerol is usually chilled and flavored in attempts to hide the real taste. Most people think it doesn't taste very good. Testing can occasionally cause nausea, sweating, lightheadedness and some other symptoms. Most test facilities ask people to arrive for the test with an empty stomach. Plan to be driven home from the testing, bring a snack and drink for after the test.

If glycerol can improve hearing why isn't it used as a treatment? Its effects are very short lived, lasting only a few hours. In addition, its taste and side effects are too negative to be dealt with daily.

REFERENCES:

Campbell, C. *Essential Audiology for Physicians*. San Diego: Singular Publishing Group, Inc., 1997.

Ferraro, J.A. and Durrant, J.D "Electrocochleography in the Evaluation of Patients with Ménière's Disease/Endolymphatic Hydrops." *Journal of the American Academy of Audiology, 17*:45–68, 2006.

Kemp, D.T. "Otoacoustic emissions, their origin in cochlear function, and use." *British Medical Bulletin, 63*:223-241, 2002.

Nguyen, L.T., Harris, J.P., and Nguyen, Q.T. "Clinical utility of electrocochleography in the diagnosis and management of Ménière's disease: AOS and ANS membership survey data." *Otology and Neurotology, 31*(3):455-459, 2010.

CHAPTER SEVENTEEN
OTHER TESTS

There are a number of other tests that might be done during the diagnostic process. None can find Ménière's; they are done to rule out other causes of the symptoms.

BLOOD TESTING

Of course there is no slam-dunk blood test to detect the presence of Ménière's disease. A few blood tests can uncover conditions like syphilis, hypothyroidism, allergies, Lyme disease, high cholesterol and autoimmune disorders capable of causing vestibular symptoms. A blood test for syphilis is important because it's still a common disease and, more important, it can be successfully treated.

A positive test is evidence that a disease is present, not that it is causing the inner ear symptoms. Some, like those for autoimmune disorders and Lyme disease, can't prove anything, but can raise suspicion.

Results of blood tests are added to all the other bits and pieces of information collected to see if evidence is mounting for a particular diagnosis.

Don't assume your doctor isn't being thorough if no exotic blood tests have been done, it could be they don't suspect anything that can be confirmed by blood tests or feel blood tests are too iffy to help (of course it's also possible they aren't being thorough).

IMAGING TESTS

Simple X-Rays of the ear are seldom done these days. Instead computerized tests like the MRI (magnetic resonance imaging) and CT (computerized tomography), capable of taking numerous "pictures," are used. None can show the insides of the inner ear or if it's working, they only show the external areas of the inner ear, the vestibulocochlear nerve and the brain.

> **SPECIAL:** If you are pregnant or might be or are trying to be, please tell both your doctor and the test facility. X-Rays can damage unborn children.

Computerized Tomography (CT)

A CT is a computerized method of taking a series of X-Rays. In the case of the ear this means looking at the temporal bone for problems like a break, wearing away of the bone, abnormal anatomy, bony defects, a tumor, cyst, or dehiscence of the superior semicircular canal.

For this test a person lays down on a table and the table is slid slowly into the CT machine where pictures are taken over a short period of time. If you are prone to claustrophobia inform the test center ahead of time.

If movement, bright lights or lying on your back stir up your symptoms plan for someone to drive you home after the test.

MRI

MRI's look at soft tissue (anything that isn't bone) using a magnetic field (instead of X-Rays). A doctor may order an MRI of the brain, the inner ear areas or both. It's generally done to look for tumors, multiple sclerosis, damage from a brain attack (stroke), hydrocephalus (water on the brain) and Arnold-Chiari malformation type I and other exotic problems. A physician usually orders this test to be absolutely sure a person doesn't have them and not because they expect to find them. A standard inner ear MRI can also help diagnose enlarged vestibular aqueduct or vestibular neuritis.

Research is underway, around the world, into techniques that would make the MRI more valuable in the diagnosis of inner ear problems, particularly visualization of endolymphatic hydrops. The research procedure includes testing before and after injecting gadolineum into the middle ear.

This test uses magnetism rather than X-Rays and has a different set of precautions, etc. to worry about. Anyone with objects in their body that can be moved with a magnet is excluded from having this test. These objects include cochlear implants, pacemakers, surgical clips and pins, metal shrapnel, or bullets. BE VERY CAREFUL ON THIS POINT—movement of metal within the body can cause injury, even death. Think at least twice before answering no. Carefully read over the literature from the testing center before going for this test. DO NOT enter the test room until certain its safe to do so.

If you are susceptible to claustrophobia discuss this with the testing center before making your appointment since the test involves being placed into a small cave-like area. An MRI in a more open machine might be possible with advance planning.

During the test you'll lay down, have your head secured so it won't move and are lowly slid inside the machine. When the machine is running it will make a loud banging noise. If they don't give you earplugs for the test insist on them. One testing sequence will be done and then an IV injection of gadolinium given and the test repeated. Gadolinium is given to help identify any abnormal growths present. Let the tech know if you have poor veins or if one arm is better than the other.

The entire testing sequence must be completed for the images to be made by the computer, don't stop the test in the middle unless it's a real emergency.

When going for the test, a person should arrange for someone to take them home in case the test procedure stirs up symptoms. Wear clothing that are comfortable and easy to remove. Don't take too many belongings along because they must be left behind in a locker.

REFERENCES:

Baloh, R.W. and Honrubia, V. *Clinical neurophysiology of the vestibular system.* Fourth edition. Oxford: Oxford University Press, 2010.

Ferri, F.F. *"Ferri's Clinical Advisor,"* Elsevier, inc, 2016.

Goebel, J.A. *Practical management of the dizzy patient. 2nd edition* Philadelphia: Lippincott William & Wilkins, 2008.

Ishiyama, G., Lopez, I.A., Sepahdari, A.R. and Ishiyama, A. "Meniere's disease: histopathology, cytochemistry, and imaging." *Annals of the New York Academy of Sciences, 1343*:49-57, 2015.

Jacobson, G. and Shepard, N. *Balance Function Assessment and Management.* San Diego: Plural Publishing, 2nd ed, 2015.

Pyykko, I., Zou, J., Poe, D., Nakashima, J. and Naganawa, S. "MRI imaging of the inner ear in Ménière's disease." *Otolaryngologic Clinics of North America, 42*:1059-1080, 2010.

CHAPTER EIGHTEEN
DIAGNOSIS: PUTTING IT ALL TOGETHER

A diagnosis may be made at any point in the information gathering and testing process. There are times when a diagnosis can be made after the history is taken and at times a firm diagnosis can not be made even after all the available information has been considered carefully including the history, symptoms, test results and the response or lack of response to a treatment.

For a diagnosis to be made the history should be consistent with Ménière's disease. Ménière's major symptoms, vertigo, hearing loss and aural fullness and/or tinnitus should be present. All the tests looking for other conditions should be negative. An improvement after starting treatment may also be used by some physicians as a sign that Ménière's disease is present.

Don't fault your doctor if they're slow to make a diagnosis. A quick, wrong, diagnosis can be more of a problem than a slow, correct one. The symptoms that are so crucial for the diagnosis don't always appear together or in rapid succession. There are cases in which years go by before the second or third symptoms appear. A rapid diagnosis is not always possible.

SECTION IV
TREATMENT

Although Ménière's disease is a chronic, incurable disease, there are a large assortment of treatments in use around the world including diet, drugs, surgery and pressure.

Treatment is one of the most controversial aspects of Ménière's disease. The following physician quotes highlight some of the problems.

"For many years the therapeutic management of this malady has been a controversial matter and one in which a confusing number of remedies have been offered, based chiefly upon the hope that they might in some manner influence some of the many hypothetical, pathologic changes which are assumed to exist.

The sum-total of these endeavors has been of little value to the patient and the causes of failure are clearly those of trial and error.

The tendency to create a disease entity by grouping a number of cases having one symptom in common is one of the temptations of medical practice. Vertigo lends itself admirably to this evil. Every conceivable form of dizziness appears to have been classified as a disease and treated as such. Failure to designate disease entities properly and apply well directed treatment has made a correlation of results impossible. There exists, therefore, no uniformity in respect to the merits of the innumerable therapeutics which have been employed.

Furstenberg, Lahmet and Lathrop, 1934

"Emotional investments create problems for all surgeons. Sometimes they have difficulty in recognizing that they need to change what they are doing. This is especially important in the management of Ménière's disease where unproven surgical procedures are often perpetuated."

Kerr, 2002

"No treatment has been found to be effective against the hearing loss, tinnitus or aural fullness through the use of a large controlled study that meets the strict criteria set up by either Cochrane or Clinical Evidence."

James and Thorpe, 2007

"Disease as devastating as Ménière's compell experimentation with new and innovative treatments. Evaluating treatment effectiveness is complicated by the exacerbating/remitting cyclic nature of Ménière's disease. In order to be a definitive study, long-term evaluations with careful contemporaneously recorded symptom diaries are required. Treatment effectiveness must be contrasted to placebo control to traditional treatments and/or to non-treatment. As in many areas of medicine not all Ménière's disease studies meet these rigorous conditions."

Hamill, 2008

Over the years treatment has been empiric, that is, based on somewhat casual observation of small numbers of people by individual doctors. Most have not necessarily been done using scientific research methods or using definitions and reporting methods recommended by large organizations such as the American Association of Otolaryngology-Head and Neck Surgery (AAOHNS). A recently published paper looking at the way research is done found randomized trials have tripled over the last two decades but their compliance with the AAOHNS guidelines and the newer recommendations by CONSORT (Consolidated standards of reporting trials) is poor.

Treatment focuses on vestibular symptoms because nothing has proven successful in stopping the progression of hearing loss and tinnitus. Instead, all three are usually addressed separately. Hearing loss can sometimes be helped with hearing amplification and if the loss is severe with cochlear implantation. Tinnitus can sometimes be helped with masking and tinnitus retraining therapy.

The hearing loss can be handled like other forms of hearing loss with hearing amplification and in extreme cases with cochlear implantation to replace the hearing. The tinnitus of Ménière's can likewise be handled like other forms of tinnitus. Masking and tinnitus retraining therapy (TRT) can be helpful to some people. If tinnitus is annoying only at night running a fan or listening to a soothing noisemaker may help.

There are many books available addressing both hearing loss and tinnitus as well as membership associations where more information can be obtained.

Many times the treatment offered has more to do with where someone lives and what their doctor believes and less about them as an individual. When talking to your doctor about treatment try to force a discussion about all the options available, not just your doctor's favorites. Hear about the pros and cons of each along with the potential side effects and problems they can cause, your doctors track record using them, recuperation time needed, the expense of each treatment and time lost from work.

Until Ménière's disease is more fully understood and a full-proof test developed, treatment will continue to be a controversial, hit or miss affair ruled more by belief than science.

The following treatment chapters are not arranged by importance but rather by increasing degree of invasiveness. The least risky treatments appear first followed by increasingly more risky.

REFERENCES:

Begg, C., Cho, M., Eastwood, S., Horton, R., Moher, D., Olkin, I., Pitkin, R., Rennie, D., Schulz, K.F., Simel, D. and Stroup, D.F. "Improving the quality of reporting of randomized controlled trials. The CONSORT statement." *Journal of the American Medical Association, 276*(8):637-639, 1996.

Furstenberg, A.C., Lashmet, F.J. and Lathrop, F. "Ménière's symptom complex: medical treatment." *Annals of Otology, Rhinology & Laryngology, 43*:1033-1046, 1934.

Hamill, T.A. "Evaluating treatments for Ménière's disease: Controversies surrounding placebo control." *Journal of the American Academy of Audiology,* 17:26-37, 2008.

James, A. and Thorp. M. "Ménière's Disease." Clinical Evidence (online), 2007:0505. http://www.ncbi.nlm.nih.gov/pmc/articles/PMC2943800/

Kerr, A.G. "Emotional investments in surgical decision making." *The Journal of Laryngology & Otology,* (116):575-579, 2002.

Sajjadi, H. and Paparella, M.M. "Ménière's Disease." *The Lancet, 372*:406-414, 2008.

Sharon, J.D., Trevino, C., Shupert, M.C. and Carey, J.P. "Treatment of Ménière's Disease." *Current Treatment Options in Neurology, 17*:14, 2015.

Syed, I and Aldren, C. "Meniere's disease: an evidence based approach to assessment and management." *International Journal of Clinical Practice, 66*:166–170, 2012.

Syed, M.I., Ilan, O., Leong, A.C., Pothier, D.D. and Rutka, J.A. "Ménière's syndrome or disease: time trends in management and quality of evidence over the last two decades." *Otology and Neurotology, 36*(8):1309-1316, 2015.

CHAPTER NINETEEN
PHYSICAL THERAPY

Vestibular rehabilitation therapy (VRT), physical therapy for vestibular disorders, is an exercise treatment for both the symptoms and poor balance of vestibular disorders. It is placed first in his section because it can be prescribed at any point during treatment; first, last or in-between.

This treatment won't get rid of the underlying cause of Ménière's disease but is particularly useful for the feeling of imbalance and the poor balance that may occur in the time between attacks. It is also very useful after some treatments such as gentamicin and vestibular nerve section.

Physical therapy was first suggested in the 1940's by a British physician. Its use didn't take off until the late 1970's. Studies have shown that this therapy has a lot of value in the right person at the right time.

This therapy can be used at any time while being treated for Ménière's disease or not used at all. The only way to find out if vestibular rehabilitation therapy will help is to give it a good try for several weeks or months.

In a perfect world this therapy would always be done by a therapist specially trained and experienced in vestibular disorders. (This is more likely to happen in an urban area). Work toward this goal is occurring on an international level with the Barany Society providing international guidelines for education in vestibular rehabilitation therapy.

GENERAL GOALS OF THERAPY

To assist the brains normal adjustment to a vestibular loss, increase reliance on the remaining vestibular information, increase reliance on vision and proprioception, improve the vestibulocular reflex, increase muscle strength, increase joint flexibility, and gain balance practice and experience.

Assist the brain's normal adjustment to a vestibular loss

When a partial loss of vestibular function occurs, the brain immediately begins the natural process of vestibular compensation. Therapy can be aimed at helping this along a bit by encouraging the use of vision and movement, two activities crucial for vestibular compensation.

Increase reliance on vestibular information

Two things can happen when an inner ear starts acting up or loses function. A person may limit their activities to avoid symptoms and/or the brain may stop the bad information from arriving in the vestibular area of the brain (due to the so-called cerebellar clamp). Both these actions lead to increased reliance on vision and proprioception. During the acute period of illness this is a good thing but if it continues too long it becomes a problem.

> The term vestibular compensation refers specifically to the chemical changes that occur in the brain allowing it to continue carrying out its balance function after a partial vestibular loss. The adjustment to total loss in each ear requires a different process called sensory substitution.

Vision is the most easily tricked of the three balance senses. If vision is used more than normal, problems misinterpreting the amount and direction of movement can occur. When vision gives information to the brain that doesn't agree with the vestibular and proprioceptive information there's a "sensory mismatch" resulting in symptoms that can be similar to seasickness. A confused brain is an unhappy brain and an unhappy brain can cause dizziness and nausea as well as vomiting.

Some people get to the point of being unable to even look at moving objects or confusing visual scenes without feeling sick. In this case exercises are prescribed to reduce the dependence on vision and improve the ability to look at movement. These exercises will include closing the eyes while standing still and walking with the eyes closed and may progress to looking at confusing or busy things as well as walking in a busy place like a mall (with the eyes open).

Overdependence on proprioception can also occur. In this case exercises begin by standing on something soft like a thick piece of foam (3" to 4" thick) and may progress to walking on highly padded carpeting or beach sand.

Increase reliance on vision and proprioception
Usually when there's a loss of nearly all-vestibular function in both ears the brain will automatically start to use vision and proprioception more for balance. This process can take a while to reach its peak with

months and sometimes a year or two needed. Exercises can be prescribed to help this process go faster and be more complete.

Improve the vestibulocular reflex

This reflex responsible for steady vision is disrupted by the loss of vestibular function or from bad vestibular information arriving in the brain. Exercises can be prescribed to help get as much use as possible from what remains of the VOR. They include things like staring at the small print on a business card taped to the wall while moving the head and can progress to watching a moving object while moving the head.

Increase muscle strength

The strength to carry out balance is just as important as the other parts of balance (joint flexibility, alertness, normal brain, normal spinal cord, experience and practice and vestibular information, vision and proprioception). Strengthening exercises can be prescribed if any areas of muscle weakness are found during the examination.

Increase joint flexibility

Joint flexibility is just as important as muscle strength and all other parts of balance. The physical therapist can recommend flexibility exercises or other therapies if joint stiffness is found during the examination, particularly in the legs.

Gain balance practice and experience

Good balance requires practice and experience at many skills in many situations. After a vestibular loss or disruption the brain may need to gain experience and practice all over again at the skills and situations needed for daily life. Some people are successful at doing this on their own and others need help to get it done.

HOW IS IT DONE?

VRT begins with an assessment by a physical therapist to determine general physical condition, balance ability, muscle strength, joint flexibility, symptoms, actions that bring symptoms on, and how much vision, proprioception and vestibular information are relied upon for balance. Assessment may also include a computerized machine. After the therapist is done with the assessment they determine what's needed, set a goal and give instructions and demonstrations of exercises to be done at home.

Unfortunately the vestibular rehabilitation therapy exercises make some people feel more off balance and nauseated for the first few days of therapy and sometimes each time new exercises are added. When undergoing vestibular rehabilitation therapy keep in mind the saying, no pain, no gain. There's no pain to these exercises but there can be a little bit of suffering that must be endured for short periods of time. They should not bring on ear fullness or pain, tinnitus and/or hearing loss. If any of these appear, therapy should be stopped immediately and the doctor who ordered the VRT notified. People who work outside the home may want to start the exercises and make changes to them on Friday evenings so they have the weekend to recuperate from any ill effects.

Taking symptom reducing drugs like meclizine or Valium or drinking alcohol probably reduces the effectiveness of the exercises. If you need any of these drugs talk to your therapist about how to proceed.

TAI CHI EXERCISE FOR BALANCE
Tai chi, a Chinese exercise regimen, has been reported by one research group to improve balance in people with vestibular disorders. Most cities and large towns have Tai chi instructors and classes.

FUTURE TRENDS:
More use of computerized systems, both in clinics and in the home itself. Because of the number of head injuries being suffered by the military on their various deployments the Department of Defense is researching and developing the Computer Assisted Rehabilitation Environment (CAREN). At some point this system might also be used in civilians with only vestibular problems.

In the civilian world, research into the use of the Nintendo Wii gaming device with balance board is underway. Research so far has been favorable. Use of the gaming device should not be undertaken without complete consideration of safety and what to do if a fall were to occur.

REFERENCES:

Balaban, C.D., Hoffer, M.E. and Gottshall, K.R. "Top-down approach to vestibular compensation: translational lessons from vestibular rehabilitation." *Brain Research, 1482*:101-111, 2012.

Blakley, B.W. "Vestibular rehabilitation on a budget." *Journal of Otolaryngology, 28(4)*:205-210, 1999.

Cawthorne, T.E. "The physiological basis for head exercises." *Journal of the Chartered Society of Physiotherapy, 29*:106, 1944.

Cawthorne, T. "Vestibular injuries." *Proceedings of the Royal Society of Medicine, 39*:270-272, 1945.

Cohen, H.S., Gottshall, K.R., Graziano, M., Malmstrom, E.M., Sharpe, M.H. and Whitney, S.L. "Barany Society Ad Hoc Committee on Vestibular Rehabiliation Therapy. International guidelines for education in vestibular rehabilitation therapy." *Journal of Vestibular Research, 21*(5):243-250, 2011.

Cooksey, F.S. "Rehabilitation in vestibular injuries." *Proceedings of the Royal Society of Medicine, 39*:273-275, 1945.

Gottshall, K.R., Hoffer, M.E., Moore, R.J. and Balough, B.J. "The role of vestibular rehabilitation in the treatment of Ménière's disease." *Otolaryngology-Head and Neck Surgery, 133*(3):326-328, 2005.

Gottshall, K.R., Topp, S.G. and Hoffer, M.E. "Early vestibular physical therapy rehabilitation for Ménière's disease." *Otolaryngological Clinics of North America, 43*(5):1113-1119, 2010.

Gottshall, K.R., Sessoms, P.H. and Bartlett, J.L. "Vestibular physical therapy intervention: utilizing a computer assisted rehabilitation environment in lieu of traditional physical therapy." *Conference Proceedings IEEE Engineering in Medicine and Biology Society*, 6141-6144, 2012.

Gottshall, K.R. and Sessoms, P.H. "Improvements in dizziness and imbalance results from using a multi disciplinary and multi sensory approach to Vestibular Physical Therapy - a case study." http://www.ncbi.nlm.nih.gov/pubmed/26300743 doi: 10.3389/fnsys.2015.00106. eCollection 2015.

Hahn, A., Sejna, I., Stolbova, K. and Cocek, A. "Visuo-vestibular biofeedback in patients with peripheral vestibular disorders." *Acta Otolaryngologica,* Supplement *545*:88-91, 2001.

Hain, T.C., Fuller, L., Weil, L. and Kotsias, J. "Effects of T'ai Chi on Balance." *Archives of Otolaryngology-Head and Neck Surgery, 125(*11):1191-1195, 1999.

Herdman, S.J. and Clendaniel, R. *Vestibular Rehabilitation.* 4th Ed. Philadelphia: F.A. Davis and Company, 2014.

Horak, F.B. "Postural compensation for vestibular loss and implications for rehabilitation." *Restorative Neurology and Neuroscience, 28*(1):57-68, 2010.

Isaacson, B.M., Swanson, T.M. and Pasquina, P.F. "The use of a computer-assisted rehabilitation environment (CAREN) for enhancing wounded warrior rehabilitation regimens." *Journal of Spinal Cord Medicine, 36*(4):296-299, 2013.

Luxon, L.M. and Davies, R.A. *Handbook of vestibular rehabilitation.* San Diego: Singular Publishing Group, Inc., 1997.

McCabe, B.F. "Labyrinthine exercises in the treatment of diseases characterized by vertigo: their physiologic basis and methodology." *Laryngoscope*, *80*:1429, 1970.

Meldrum, D., Glennon, A., Herdman, S., Murray, D. and McConn-Walsh, R. "Virtual reality rehabilitation of balance: assessment of the usability of the Nintendo Wii(®) Fit Plus." *Disability Rehabilitation Assistive Technology*, *7*(3):205-210, 2012.

Shepard, N.T. and Jacobson, G.P. *Balance Function Assessment and Management. San Diego, CA:* Plural Publishing, 2008.

Sparrer, I., Duong Dinh, T.A., Ilgner, J. and Westhofen, M. "Vestibular rehabilitation using the Nintendo® Wii Balance Board -- a user-friendly alternative for central nervous compensation." *Acta Otolaryngologica*, *133*(3):239-245, 2013.

Telian, S.A. and Shepard, N.T. "Update on vestibular rehabilitation therapy." *Otolaryngologic Clinics of North America*, 29:357-371, 1996.

CHAPTER TWENTY
DIET

Diet changes have been recommended to people with the Ménière's disease diagnosis going back to 1934 when Furstenberg and his colleagues saw improvement in their small group of patients eating the diet and taking a diuretic. This idea received a boost in 1938 with the discovery of endolymphatic hydrops.

Note: This was a small study with no control group, that is, no group of people with Ménière's disease being observed but not receiving the treatment. This evidence is not strong compared to a study done with a large group of people and a control group. None of the diets or diet supplements have had large, controlled studies done, all are based on the experience of the doctor prescribing them.

There are a number of diets recommended by physicians based on their belief of what causes Ménière's disease and/or its symptoms. Dietary regimens are part of the most common initial treatment approach to Ménière's disease in the U.S. Diet changes and the use of various diet supplements will not get rid of the underlying disease, at best they may reduce the number, frequency or severity of vertigo attacks, and perhaps decrease in the pressure and tinnitus.

There's no way to predict ahead of time if a diet change will help. The only way to find out is through trial and error under a doctor's supervision. None of these diet changes have been studied with large groups compared to a control group.

DIETS
Low Salt
Doctors who feel too much endolymph is being produced prescribe a low-sodium diet. If the diet doesn't work after a few weeks a diet even lower in sodium might be suggested.

Following a low sodium diet is difficult because it goes well beyond not using the saltshaker. Processed, ready made, fast food and restaurant foods are loaded with sodium and must be taken into account. A successful low sodium diet depends upon the use of fresh or frozen fruits, vegetables, meat, and fish and paying a lot of attention to detail as well as determination.

Caffeine

A low caffeine diet is thought, by the doctors recommending it, to improve circulation to the inner ear and within the inner ear.

Caffeine occurs naturally in chocolate (dark or semi-sweet has the most), coffee and all colors of tea, Coca-cola, Pepsi-cola and other cola's. It's added to a number of drinks such as Mountain Dew, Sunkist Orange and Barq's Root beer and is an ingredient in some over-the-counter anti-sleeping aids as well as many energy drinks. Read all labels carefully when trying to avoid caffeine.

The good news is that coffee, tea, coca-cola and pepsi-cola are all available in "no caffeine added" versions.

Allergy

A food elimination diet may be prescribed when an allergy is suspected. An elimination diet is really used as a diagnostic test rather than as a treatment. A symptom diary is kept while various foods are not eaten or eliminated from the diet. If symptoms improve or go away when a food has been stopped it's assumed the eliminated food was the problem and it's then avoided in the future. If a gluten allergy is suspected a gluten free diet may be suggested.

In addition to the food elimination diet there's the rotating diet in which foods a person is allergic to are eaten only every 5 days or so.

Migraine

Some doctors prescribe a migraine diet when they feel there is a relationship between migraine and Ménière's disease. Food doesn't cause migraines to begin but a number of different foods are thought to bring on attacks in some people who suffer from migraines. Simply not eating those foods can help stop attacks. These foods include: Red wine, aged cheese (like cheddar), chocolate, citrus fruits and foods containing monosodium glutamate (MSG), nitrate or aspartame (artificial sweetener).

Carbohydrate

Doctors who feel general fluctuations in body fluids cause symptoms may suggest limiting the simple carbohydrate foods and candies in the diet along with spreading out meals over the entire day.

DIET SUPPLEMENTS
Diet supplements including Lipoflavonoids and ginger are sometimes recommended by doctors.

Lipoflavonoids
This diet supplement appears in the medical literature in both 1965 and 1970. The physicians studying it found some of their patients had improvements in vertigo and hearing when taking it. None of the studies were large and/or controlled. In 2016 the one company producing this supplement was asked by the National Advertising Review Board to stop claiming it can help either tinnitus or Ménière's disease.

Lipoflavonoids contain eriodictyol, glycoside (found naturally in lemon peel) and the following vitamins: vitamin B6 and B12 (B complex), vitamin C, niacin, riboflavin, thiamine, choline, inositol and pantothenic acid.

Although classified as a dietary supplement this drug is not without potential dangers. It may interfere with other drugs such as ibuprofen, diuretics and blood pressure medications. This should only be taken under the supervision of a physician.

Ginger
Although not studied in Ménière's disease, ginger has been found useful to some people suffering from nausea and vomiting. Studies include pregnant woman with morning sickness and some individuals undergoing chemotherapy for cancer.

EVIDENCE
There are no large, well-controlled studies supporting the use of any of these diet changes but there are many individual stories of their helpfulness. There's no way to predict ahead of time if a diet change will help. The only way to find out is through trial and error under a doctor's supervision. It can take weeks to see if a diet change helps.

REFERENCES:

Creston, J.E., Gillespie, M.R. and Larson, A.L. "Bioflavonoid Therapy in Sensorineural Hearing Loss: A Double Blind Study," *Archives of Otolaryngology*, *82*(2):159-165, 1965.

Furstenberg, A.C., Lashmet, F.J. and Lathrop, F. "Ménière's symptom complex: medical treatment." *Annals of Otology, Rhinology & Laryngology*, *43*:1033-1046, 1934.

Goffin, F.B. "Lipoflavonoids in Ménière's disease." *Eye, Ear, Nose and Throat Monthly*, *49*(6):290-291,1970.

Luxford, E., Berliner, K., Lee, J. and Luxford, W.M. "Dietary modification as adjunct treatment in Ménière's disease: patient willingness and ability to comply." *Otology and Neurotology*, *34*(8):1438-1443, 2013.

NARB Recommends Clarion Brands Modify, Discontinue Claims That Dietary Supplement 'Lipo-Flavonoid Plus' Substantially Reduces, Eliminates Tinnitus http://www.asrcreviews.org/ NY,NY April 12, 2016.

Santos, P.M., Hall, R.A., Snyder, J.M., Hughes, L.F. and Dobie, R.A. "Diuretic and diet effect on Ménière's Disease Evaluated by the 1985 Committee on Hearing and Equilibrium Guidelines." *Otolaryngology-Head and Neck Surgery*, *109*(4):680-689, 1993.

Slattery, W.H. and Fayad, J.N. "Medical treatment of Meniere's disease." *Otolaryngologic Clinics of North America, 30*(6): 1027-1037, 1997.

Smith, W.K., Sankar, V. and Pfleiderer, A.G. "A national survey amongst UK otolaryngologists regarding treatment of Ménière's disease." *Journal of Laryngology and Otology*, *119*(2):102-105, 2000.

CHAPTER TWENTY-ONE
DRUGS OVERVIEW

Drugs are routinely used around the world for Ménière's disease. Unfortunately no drug treatment has been shown to stop or reverse the damage of the disease. Most drugs in use instead target the symptoms and lost function.

Not every doctor has the same drug treatment approach. What they use depends upon their belief about Ménière's disease and what their experience has been with the different drugs available. Some doctors will prescribe one drug while others use many drugs in the so-called shotgun approach. This approach probably has the best chance of helping but if it is successful there's no way to know which drug or combination of drugs did the trick.

In the U.S. diuretics are the most commonly used medicines given in an effort to reduce inner ear fluid pressure. Symptom blockers are used to lessen the nausea, vomiting, motion sickness and spinning. Sometimes steroids are used in an attempt to reduce inflammation. Drugs thought to enhance inner ear circulation may be given. Anti-immune system drugs like steroids and Enbrel may be used if an immune system attack on the ear is suspected. Drugs may also be used for depression, anxiety, and allergies. A drug called gentamicin is used on occasion to intentionally damage the inner ear.

Drugs can be placed into the blood stream to travel through the body eventually reaching the area where they are needed. They can be injected directly into the blood stream via a vein, injected into a muscle, swallowed or given as a suppository. Drugs can be placed directly into the ear. They can't be injected directly into the inner ear but can be placed into the middle ear and travel into the inner ear through the oval and round windows

CHAPTER TWENTY-TWO
DIURETICS

For decades diuretics, commonly known as water pills, have been widely prescribed for Ménière's disease. In the U.S. they are the first or second treatment option offered by 72.8% of ear specialists in one study. In the U.K. a 2005 survey of otolaryngologists found 63% prescribing diuretics in the belief they reduce the number and/or severity of vertigo attacks by decreasing the amount of endolymph fluid, reducing the sodium in the inner ear or stopping fluid fluctuations in the inner ear.

Surprisingly there's been very little research to support their use. In the words of the *Cochrane Database of Systematic Reviews* "there is insufficient good evidence of the effect of diuretics on vertigo, hearing loss, tinnitus or aural fullness in clearly defined Ménière's disease." *Clinical Evidence* 2005 also found no evidence diuretics affect disease progression.

A few human studies have been done but were small, of short length and didn't compare the treatment group to a group receiving no treatment. They are summarized below:

- 33 people were given the diuretic Dyazide for a period of time and a placebo was also given to the same people for the same amount of time. Nobody experienced improvement in hearing or tinnitus while 17 of the 33 did have an improvement in vertigo while on Dyazide. Three participants had vertigo improvement while on the placebo and 13 felt no difference between the diuretic and placebo. This works out to an improvement rate of just over 50% for those on the diuretic.

- For five years, researchers followed 79 people on daily chlorthalidone, 42 people on daily acetazolamide and 71 treated intermittently when their symptoms increased. They found that 2 to 6 weeks into treatment the hearing loss typically improved for those on the diuretics but there was no difference between the groups at the end of 5 or more years.

- 54 people were treated with diuretics and a low-salt diet for two years. 79% had complete or substantial control of vertigo, 19% no real change, 2% became worse. Hearing improved in 35%, didn't change in 29%, got worse in 22% and could not be classified in 14%.

Despite this some people do seem to be helped by diuretics. Because they are relatively inexpensive, easy to use and have less risk then many other treatments, diuretics have become a first line treatment for Ménière's Disease.

All diuretics work by manipulating chemicals in the kidneys causing more water to leave the entire body in the urine. All diuretics remove sodium from the body, many remove potassium, a few hang on to the potassium and some change other chemicals.

In the U.S., the diuretic most commonly used for Ménière's disease is hydrochorothiazide (HCTZ) alone or in combination with triamterene. The drug combination of HCTZ and triamterene is marketed as the generic HCTZ/triamterene and under the names Dyazide and Maxzide in the US, Apo-Triazide, Novo-Triamzide and Nu-Triazide in Canada. HCTZ alone causes loss of potassium that must be replaced through the diet and with a potassium supplement. When administered as the combination drug potassium loss is usually not a problem, however both low and high potassium levels are possible.

Although diuretics are given to reduce sodium it must be understood sodium is a mineral needed for proper body function. It participates in water balance and movement, fluid pressure regulation, nerve function, muscle function, and it helps transport glucose and other nutrients within the body. Sodium levels must be kept within certain limits for our survival. Both too little and too much create problems. Diuretics aren't used to rid the body of all sodium, but to keep the sodium level at the lower end of normal and at a steady amount, i.e. not fluctuating.

If placed on a diuretic by your specialist notify your GP/PCP. Find out how much water to drink daily, if a potassium based salt substitute can be used, how often sodium and potassium levels should be checked and what symptoms/changes to report. Do not stop drinking fluids while taking diuretics unless your specialist has instructed you to do this and your PCP has agreed you won't be harmed.

Medical Hypothesis in 2011 printed a question about their safety. The hypothesis put forward: A diuretic might lower blood pressure and thereby interfere with the blood supply of the inner ear, possibly causing permanent damage. This is a hypothesis or educated guess based on their knowledge, not based on research. The use of diuretics is also a hypothesis.

Reduction in potassium is sometimes an unintended consequence of diuretic use. Potassium is used throughout the body to send nerve messages and contract muscles, helps in building proteins, converts glucose to glycogen, helps regulate acid/base balance, builds muscle and is used in the inner ear for both hearing and vestibular function. It must be present in the right amount for the body to work correctly. The potassium and sodium levels should be checked routinely when diuretics are taken whether or not the diuretic is the potassium losing type.

Not everyone can tolerate diuretics. They cause a body-wide reduction in water and chemicals that may cause dehydration, faintness, low blood pressure, muscle weakness/spasms, headaches, fatigue and more. The symptoms of sodium and potassium changes are non-specific; there is nothing special about them. The only way to diagnose abnormally high or low sodium and potassium levels is a blood test, the serum electrolyte test.

If your Ménière's symptoms don't improve in three or four months on a diuretic have a discussion with your specialist about using another diuretic or stopping diuretic therapy. There isn't much sense taking a drug with body-wide effects that isn't working.

REFERENCES:

Clyde, J.W., Oberman, B.S. and Isildok. T.L. "Current management practices in Meniere's Disease." *Otology and Neurotology*, 38(6):159-167, 2017.

Crowson, M.G., Patik, A. and Tucci, D.L. "A systematic review of diuretics in the medical management of Meniere's Disease." *Otolaryngology-Head and Neck Surgery*, 154(5):824-834, 2016.

Furstenberg, A.C., Lashmet, F.J. and Lathrop, F. "Ménière's symptom complex: medical treatment." *Annals of Otology, Rhinology & Laryngology*, 43:1033-1046, 1934.

James, A.L. and Thorp, M.A. "Meniere's disease." BMJ *Clinical Evidence* 2007:0505.

Pirodda, A., Ferri, G.G., Raimondi, M.C. and Borghi, C. "Diuretics in Meniere disease: a therapy or a potential cause of harm?" *Medical Hypotheses*, 77(5):869-871, 2011.

Smith, W.K., Sankar, V. and Pfleiderer, A.G. "A national survey amongst UK otolaryngologists regarding the treatment of Ménière's disease." *Journal of Laryngology and Otology*, 119(2):102-105, 2005.

van Deelen, G.W. and Huizing, E.H. "Use of a diuretic (Dyazide) in the treatment of Meniere's disease: a double-blind cross-over placebo-controlled study." *Journal for Oto-Rhino-Laryngology and its Related Specialties*, 48: 287-292, 1986.

Thirlwall, A.S. and Kundu, S. "Diuretics for Ménière's disease or syndrome." *Cochrane Database Systematic Review*, issue 3 Art. No.:CD003599. DOI 10.1002/14651858, CD003599. Pbb2.

CHAPTER TWENTY-THREE
ANTI-SYMPTOM DRUGS: INSIDE THE US

Although they can't stop the Ménière's disease, drugs can block symptoms, at least to some degree. If they cover up vestibular symptoms they're called vestibular suppressants and if they reduce nausea and vomiting they're called anti-emetics.

Symptom blockers do have some drawbacks:

- Vestibular suppressants and/or anti-emetics interfere with vestibular tests.

- Suppressants also interfere with the normal way the body adapts to the loss of vestibular function.

- The drowsiness from some can lead to increased danger driving and operating machinery and power tools (don't climb ladders or anything else requiring good balance and coordination while under the effect of these drugs).

- In exchange for less vestibular symptoms, balance function may worsen.

- They can cause drowsiness and blurred vision and make a person feel quite a bit worse (which may be mistaken for worsening of the vestibular problem).

- Alcohol must be avoided when taking many of these drugs.

- Memory and thought may be affected.

- Meclizine, cyclizine, dimenhydrinate and promethazine can interfere with allergy testing.

Some vestibular suppressants, like meclizine and dimenhydrinate, can be purchased over-the-counter, others must be prescribed. Many drugs from a number of drug classes are available.

MECLIZINE
Meclizine is widely used in Ménière's disease and other vestibular disorders to stop nausea/vomiting and calm the vestibular system. It is also sold over the counter as an antimotion sickness medication.

Other names: Bonine, Antivert, Dramamine Less Drowsy, Verticalm, Zentrip.

How it comes: Regular tablet and as a chewable tablet, the chewable can also be swallowed whole.

Effects: Meclizine is an H-1 antihistamine and anticholinergic with sedative and antivomiting effects. Used to prevent motion sickness, prevent or stop nausea/vomiting, and can also be used for allergies.

How it is taken: For an attack; around the clock for a period of time.

Timing: Begins to work in about an hour. Half the drug is gone in about 6 hours.

Cautions: Use with caution in people over 65 and particularly anyone with dementia, glaucoma, enlarged prostate, urinary tract blockage or asthma. If you are pregnant or trying to get pregnant this drug is thought to be safe.

Possible side effects: Drowsiness, dry mouth, sedation.

Interactions: The sedation and sleepiness can be increased by alcohol, barbiturates and other sedatives, narcotics, tranquilizers, sleeping aids and any other drugs that act in the brain including marijuana, cocaine and other illegal drugs.

Evidence for its use: No studies of its use in Ménière's disease have been done but the drug has been around for a long time and has a low rate of side effects. The anti-nausea/vomiting and anti-motion sickness properties are well known.

DIMENHYDRINATE

Dimenhydrinate is widely used in Ménière's disease, other vestibular disorders and seasickness to stop nausea/vomiting and calm the vestibular system. It is sold over the counter as an anti-motion sickness medication. Its technical drug category is H1 antihistamine, it blocks histamine in the vestibular and vomiting brain centers.

Effects: Has sedative and anti-vomiting effects. Used to prevent motion sickness, prevent or stop nausea/vomiting, and can also be used for allergies.

Other names: Dramamine Original.

How it comes: Tablet and can be given by injection in a hospital.

How it is taken: For an attack; around the clock for a period of time.

Other names: Dramamine, Dramamine chewable, Gravol (Canada), Dimetabs, Dinate (Canada).

Timing: Tablets work in 15 to 30 minutes, lasts 3-6 hours. Injections work in 20-30 minutes.

Possible side effects: Sleepiness, dizziness, blurred vision, headache, hyperactivity (esp. kids), ringing in the ears, dry mouth/nose/throat, fast/pounding/irregular heartbeat, constipation, poor appetite, skin rash.

Cautions: DO NOT DRIVE A CAR, OPERATE MACHINERY, CLIMB A LADDER or any other activity that would be affected by drowsiness. Tell your doctor if you have any of the following: Asthma, shortness of breath, chronic bronchitis, emphysema, enlarged prostate, glaucoma, phenylketonuria (concern with chewable form), pregnancy, nursing mothers.

Interactions: Alcohol, sedatives, strong pain relievers, sleeping pills, antidepressive drugs, muscle relaxants and tranquilizers can increase the drowsiness.

Evidence for its use: No studies of its use in Ménière's disease have been done but the drug has been around for a long time and has a low rate of side effects. The anti-nausea/vomiting and anti-motion sickness properties are well known.

PROMETHAZINE

This drug is sometimes used in Ménière's disease to stop vomiting and calm the vestibular system. It differs from other anti-motion sickness / anti-vomiting drugs because it is also available as a suppository and can be used successfully during a time of active vomiting.

Other names: Promethegan, Phenergan.

Effects: Promethazine is an H1 receptor blocking agent or antihistamine with sedative and anti-vomiting effects. Used to prevent motion sickness, prevent or stop nausea/vomiting, and can also be used for allergies.

Comes as: Tablets, syrup and suppositories. Can be injected as well.

Timing: Begins to work in about 20 minutes after taking a pill and generally last four to six hours, although it could last as long as 12 hours.
Possible side effects: Dizziness, drowsiness, anxiety, blurred vision, dry

---

Akathisia – The inability to sit still.

Athetosis – Constant, slow, involuntary movement of the fingers, toes, hands and feet in which they are placed palm up and then palm down.

Hemiballism – Involuntary movement of the arm and leg on one side of the body that looks like jerking.

Any drug capable of causing extrapyramidal symptoms should not be taken regularly for long periods of time.

---

mouth, stuffy nose, ringing in the ears, weight gain, hand and feet swelling, impotence, sleep disturbance, trouble having a orgasm, constipation, loss of coordination, nervousness, restlessness, itching, extrapyramidal symptoms (see table).

Interactions: MAO antidepressants (Monoamine oxidase inhibitors). Mental impairment is increased by alcohol, barbiturates and other sedatives, narcotics, tricyclic antidepressants, tranquilizers, sleeping aids.

Cautions: CHILDREN TWO AND UNDER SHOULD NOT TAKE THIS DRUG. Tell your doctor if you have any of the following: Asthma, chronic obstructive pulmonary disease, sleep apnea, sulfite allergy, seizures, weak immune system, glaucoma, enlarged prostate, problems with urination, stomach ulcer, heart disease, high blood pressure, liver disease, pheochromocytoma, hypocalcemia, pregnancy or trying to get pregnant.

142

Evidence for its use: This is an older drug that has been in use for nausea and vomiting a long time, there is no controversy about its general use. There are no studies looking at its use in Ménière's disease. During the period of shuttle space flight promethazine was routinely given to astronauts to treat space sickness (similar to motion sickness) with 60% reporting it helped.

ONDANSETRON

Ondansetron is approved for the nausea and vomiting of surgery, chemotherapy and radiation therapy and is used on occasion for the nausea and vomiting of vestibular disorders. Ondansetron is an expensive drug but may help if other, cheaper, drugs aren't working.

Other names: Zofran.

Effects: It's a member of the newer selective serotonin 5-HT3 receptor antagonist drug group that blocks the action of serotonin. It stops vomiting signals that are made by the release of serotonin.

Comes as: Tablet, IV infusion, rectal suppository.

Timing: Pills require 30 to 120 minutes to reach their maximum, 50% of the drug is gone from the body in 3 to 5 hours.

Possible side effects: Can impair thought and reactions but less than other anti-vomiting drugs, don't drive or any other activities that require alertness, diarrhea, lightheadedness, rash, blurred vision, dizziness, constipation, headache.

Interactions: Apomorphine, tramadol, dilantin, tegretol rifadin with MAO inhibitors, SSRI inhibitors such as fluoxetine (Prozac) paroxetine (paxil) or sertraline (Zoloft).

Caution: Pregnancy, heart rhythm problem such as long QT syndrome. Some types of Ondansetron, like the orally disintegrating tablets, may contain phenylketonuria.

Evidence for its use: This drug has been in use for the vomiting of surgery, chemotherapy and radiation for more than twenty years. No studies have been done on its use in Ménière's disease, but there is one study of its use in vestibular neuritis that was favourable.

BENZODIAZEPINES

Drugs of the benzodiazepine family may be prescribed to help block abnormal movement sensations such as vertigo. These drugs can also reduce muscle tension, anxiety and seizure activity. Xanax also reduces tinnitus in some people.

Effects: They are thought to work in the brain and might do so by an action on GABA, one of the brain neurotransmitters.

Comes as: Valium, Klonopin, Xanax.

Timing (pill form): Starts working in an hour or two, how long it remains in the body depends upon which benzodiazepine, half of Valium is gone in 20 to 50 hours and Xanax in 6 to 20 hours.

Possible side effects: Drowsiness. Their major drawback is addiction. There's a 50% chance of having withdrawal symptoms when the drug is stopped after 8 or more months but they can also appear when the drug has been used as little as 4 to 6 weeks. Benzodiazepines can also lead to depression and trouble thinking.

Interactions: Alcohol, sedatives, strong pain relievers, sleeping pills, antidepressive drugs, muscle relaxants and tranquilizers can increase the drowsiness.

Evidence for its use: Although in wide use no randomized clinical trials for their use has been done. Their use is based on the individual experience of different doctors.

Stopping or reducing the dosage of these drugs leads to the following situations in some people:

- *Withdrawal* – The start of new symptoms as a result of stopping a drug.
- *Relapse* – A gradual return of the original symptoms.
- *Rebound* – A return of the original symptoms at a more intense level.

SEROTONIN MANIPULATING DRUGS

Drugs of both the tricyclic antidepressant family and the SSRI's (selective serotonin reuptake inhibitors) can lessen vestibular symptoms in some people as well as reduce depression and anxiety.

Effects: How they work is unknown but most theories revolve around an affect on neurotransmitters, the chemicals that carry on the work of the nervous system.

Comes as:
Tricyclics: Amitriptyline (Elavil), imipramine (Tofranil), nortriptyline (Pamelor) and desipramine (Norpramine).

SSRI's: Prozac (fluoxetine), Zoloft (sertraline), Paxil (paroxetine), Luvox (fluvoxamine) and Celexa (citalopram).

Timing: These drugs work very slowly, days to a week or two may be needed for any effect to take place.

Interactions: Alcohol, sedatives, warfarin blood thinner, diuretics, beta-blockers, digoxin, antiarrythmia drugs and many others. Discuss all your drugs with your physician before taking this drug, have all of your drug prescriptions filled at the same pharmacy so your pharmacist can be aware as well.

Caution: Stopping these drugs suddenly can lead to rebound symptoms, the return of prior symptoms at a stronger level. Some people also experience trouble with balance and/or develop new vestibular symptoms.

Evidence for their use: Widely used for depression. There are some studies indicating these are useful in a number of vestibular problems including vestbular migraine and Ménière's disease.

GINGER

This food substance is well known to help decrease the nausea and vomiting of motion sickness, pregnancy, chemotherapy and surgery, in some people. It's a food that can be eaten in many ways such as ginger ale, ginger snap cookies, pickled ginger or as a capsule.

Ginger works in the stomach rather than in the brain so there's no drowsiness, or other disturbing side effects from the drug.

Because this is a food, very little data is available about effectiveness and possible interactions with drugs.

Interaction: Nifedipine

Timing: Thought to work rapidly.

Evidence for its use: There are a few reports from small studies showing it helps, at times. No large randomized, controlled studies have been done.

GETTING MORE DRUG INFORMATION

Start with your doctor and pharmacist when you need more information about drugs. If they aren't giving you enough information you have three options, stop searching for more information, change to a doctor who will give you the information you want or do your own work.

REFERENCES:

http://www.nlm.nih.gov/medlineplus/druginfo/meds/a682548.html
http://www.nhs.uk/medicine-guides/pages/MedicineOverview.aspx?condition=Sedation&medicine=promethazine

Bailey, K.P "Selective serotonin reuptake inhibitor discontinuation syndrome." *Journal of Psychosocial Nursing, 40*(12):12-18, 2002.

Barratt, M.R. and Pool, S. L. *Principles of Clinical Medicine for Space Flight.* New York: Springer, 2008.

Dyhrfjeld-Johnsen, J., Gaboyard-Niay, S., Broussy, A., Saleur, A., Brugeaud, A. and Chabbert, C. "Ondansetron reduces lasting vestibular deficits in a model of severe peripheral excitotoxic injury." *Journal of Vestibular Research, 23*(3):177-186, 2013.

Gilbert, C., Mazzotta, P., Loebstein, R. and Koren, G. "Fetal safety of drugs used in the treatment of allergic rhinitis: a critical review." *Drug Safety, 28*(8):707-719, 2005.

Goto, F., Tsutsumi, T. and Ogawa, K. "Successful treatment of relapsed Ménière's disease using selective serotonin reuptake inhibitors: A report of three cases." *Experimental Therapeutic Medicine, 7*(2):488-490, 2014.

Grøntved, A. and Hentzer, E. "Vertigo-reducing effect of ginger root. A controlled clinical study." *ORL J Otorhinolaryngol Related Specialties, 48*(5):282-286, 1986.

Horii, A., Mitani, K., Kitahara, T., Uno, A., Takeda, N. and Kubo, T. "Paroxetine, a selective serotonin reuptake inhibitor, reduces depressive symptoms and subjective handicaps in patients with dizziness." *Otology and Neurotology, 25*(4):536-543, 2004.

Katzung, B.G., Masters, S.B. and Trevor, A.J. *Basic & clinical pharmacology.* New York: McGraw-Hill Medical, 2012.

Roila, F. and Del Favero, A. "Ondonsetron." *Clinical Pharmacokinetetics, .29*(2):95-109, 1995.

Simon, N.M., Parker, S.W., Wernick-Robinson, M., Oppenheimer, J.E., Hoge, E.A.,Worthington, J.J., Korbly, N.B. and Pollack, M.H. "Fluoxetine for vestibular dysfunction and anxiety: a prospective pilot study." *Psychosomatics 46*(4):334-339, 2005.

Staab, J.P., Ruckenstein, M.J. and Amsterdam, J.D. "A prospective trial of sertraline for chronic subjective dizziness." *Laryngoscope, 114*(9):1637-1641, 2004.

Qiu, J.X., Zhou, Z.W., He, Z.X., Zhang, X·, Zhou, S.F. and Zhu, S. "Estimation of the binding modes with important human cytochrome P450 enzymes, drug interaction potential, pharmacokinetics, and hepatotoxicity of ginger components using molecular docking, computational, and pharmacokinetic modeling studies." *Drug Design Development and Therapy, 16*(9):841-866, 2015.

Venail, F., Biboulet, R., Mondain, M. and Uziel A. "A protective effect of 5-HT3 antagonist against vestibular deficit? Metoclopramide versus ondansetron at the early stage of vestibular neuritis: a pilot study." *European Annals of Otorhinolaryngology, Head and Neck Disease, 129*(2):65-68, 2012.

CHAPTER TWENTY-FOUR
ANTI-SYMPTOM DRUGS: OUTSIDE US

This chapter describes three anti-symptom drugs in wide use outside the US; Betahistine, Cinnarizine and Flunarizine.

BETAHISTINE DIHYDROCHLORIDE
Betahistine dihydrochloride is in wide spread use throughout the world. It is a mainstay of treatment in the UK with a reported 94% of ENT's prescribing it to their patients with Ménière's disease. It does NOT cause drowsiness and has a low incidence of side effects. In the UK it is also widely used for non-Ménière's vertigo as well (113,000 prescriptions are filled monthly but only around 28,224 people have a Ménière's disease diagnosis).

Other names: Serc, Betaserc, Hiserk, Veserc.

Effects: Originally the theory of its effect was vasodilatation in the circulation of the inner ear. Now the drug is considered a central nervous system drug. It is a histamine H3 receptor agonist meaning it increases the amounts of the chemicals histamine, acetylcholine, norepinephrine and serotonin in some areas of the body. It's thought, by those prescribing it, to increase serotonin and decrease vertigo and nausea by inhibiting the vestibular nuclei in the brain. Recent research has found sites in the endolymphatic sac where betahistine might work.

Timing: The half-life is 3-4 hours, that is, half the drug is gone from the body within 3-4 hours.

Cautions: Not to be used in children, people with peptic ulcer, asthma, allergic skin conditions or pheochromocytoma; during pregnancy (or while trying to become pregnant) or while breastfeeding. The tablets should be taken with meals.

Possible side effects: Skin irritations, stomach upsets, dizziness, fast heartbeat, headache, difficulty sleeping, chest tightness, and nausea.

Interactions: Antihistamines, selegiline, tricyclic antidepressants such as elavil and pamelor, monoamine oxidase inhibitor type antidepressants.

Evidence for its use: As with most treatments the evidence is mixed.

Many small studies claiming its usefulness exist but the 2010 Cochrane Database of Systematic Reviews concluded there was insufficient evidence to determine whether betahistine had any effect on Ménière's disease. The entire Cochrane article can be accessed at: http://onlinelibrary.wiley.com/doi/10.1002/14651858.CD001873/full Clinical Evidence by the British Medical Journal also concluded there is no good evidence.

A 2016 German study conducted @ 14 different centers using 221 people found no difference in the number of attacks in people on low dose betahistamine, high dose betahistine and placebo.

On the other hand a 2014 paper looked at several studies and concludes, "Our meta-analysis supports the therapeutic benefit of betahistine on vertiginous symptoms in both Ménière's disease and vestibular vertigo."

An MRI study found Betahistine had no effect on the Endolymphatic hydrops of the 6 patients studied.

WHY ISN'T BETHISTINE (SERC) MARKETED IN THE US?
In the US it was approved and used between 1966 and 1972. The approval was removed after discrepancies and untruths were found in the drug study the approval had depended upon. The pharmaceutical company, Unimed, was given the opportunity to contest this action and failed to do so in a court appeal. The F.D.A. also took the further step of looking at current studies for evidence of the drugs usefulness in Ménière's disease before withdrawing approval in December of 1972.

All the steps taken by the F.D.A. can be found in the Federal Register as noted in the reference list below. The F.D.A. did not find the drug to be harmful, it just found there was no longer any evidence of it's effectiveness in Ménière's disease, once the drug study was invalidated.

In 1999 betahistine was added to the F.D.A.'s Bulks Compounding List. With a U.S. doctors prescription someone with Ménière's disease living in the U.S. can obtain the drug from a compounding pharmacy. This type pharmacy makes the drug onsite. The law regulating this area specifically states a compounding pharmacy cannot advertise on behalf of a specific drug so anyone who wants it has to do the work to find a pharmacy able to make betahistine.

Betahistine can also be brought back from overseas in small amounts. Carrying more than a three-month supply on your person may raise alarms with customs officers. A doctor's prescription is also needed when attempting to get a supply from outside the U.S., usually from a doctor in the overseas location.

REFERENCES:

Adrian, C., Fisher, C.S., Wagner, J., Gurkov, R., Mansman, U. Strupp, M. "Efficacy and safety of betahistine treatment in patients with Meniere's disease: primary results of a long-term, multicentre, doubleblind, randomized, placebo controlled, dose defining trial (BEME trial)." *British Medical Journal, 352*:h6816, 2016.

Federal Register vol 33(138) July 17 1968 docket no fdc-d-111 ND NO 14-241 Unimed, Inc Serc Tablets; Notice of opportunity for hearing.

Federal Register, vol 35 no 222 Nov 14 1970 docket no fdc0d0111 nda 14-241 serc tablet; notice of order withdrawing approval of new-drug application and refusal to approve all supplements.

Gürkov, R., Flatz, W., Keeser, D., Strupp, M., Ertl-Wagner, B. and Krause E. "Effect of standard-dose Betahistine on endolymphatic hydrops: an MRI pilot study." *European Archives of Otorhinolaryngology, 270*(4):1231-1235, 2013.

Harcourt, J., Barraclough, K. and Bronstein, A.M. "Ménière's disease." *British Medical Journal, 349*:6544, 2014.

James, A. L. and Burton, M.J. "Betahistine for Meniere's disease or syndrome" *Cochrane Database* Syst Rev 1: CD001873. Updated in 2009 -- Cochrane database review, 2001.

Moller, M.N., Kirkeby, S., Vikesa, J., Nielson, F.C. and Caye-Thomasen. "Expression of histamine receptors in the human Endolymphatic sac: the molecular rationale for betahistine use in Ménière's disease." *European Archives of Otorhinolaryngology, DOI 10.1007/s00405-015-3731-5.*

Nauta, J.J. "Meta-analysis of clinical studies with betahistine in Ménière's disease and vestibular vertigo." *European Archives of Otorhinolaryngology, 271*(5):887-897, 2014.

Phillips, J.S. and Prinsley, P.R. "Prescribing practices for betahistine." *British Journal of Clinical Pharmacology, 65*(4):470-471, 2008.

Redon, C.L., Lopez, C., Bernard-Demanze, L., Dumitrescu, M., Magnan, J., Lacour, M. and Borel, L. "Betahistine treatment improves the recovery of static symptoms in patients with unilateral vestibular loss." *Journal of Clinical Pharmacology, 51*(4):538-548, 2011.

Smith, W.K., Sankar, V. and Pfleiderer, A.G. "A national survey amongst UK otolaryngologists regarding the treatment of Meniere's disease." *Laryngology and Otology, 119*(2):102-105, 2005.

CINNARIZINE

Cinnarizine is in widespread use for both motion sickness and Ménière's disease in the UK, Europe and some areas of Asia and South America. This drug is both an antihistamine and a mild calcium channel blocker. It is available by both prescription and over the counter without a prescription.

Other names include: Mylan Travel Sickness, Stugeron, Arlevert (when Cinnarizine is combined with dimenhydrinate)

Timing: This drug begins to work in 30 minutes and its affects last about 8 hours.

Possible side effects: Drowsiness, tiredness, blurred vision, indigestion, feeling sick, weight gain, headache, dry mouth, upset stomach, indigestion, dry mouth, increased sweating, itchy skin bumps, rash, jaundice, Parkinsonism, jerky or slow movements, muscle stiffness, trembling, restless, twitching or unusual movements of the tongue, face, mouth, jaw or throat, rolling of the eyes, depression, increased saliva.

Cautions: Contains lactose and sucrose and should be used with caution in the elderly, do not use if pregnant or breastfeeding.

Interactions: Alcohol may increase the drowsiness, should not take with MAO inhibitors, a type of antidepressant, or with tricyclic antidepressants. Check with your doctor before using this drug if you have: Liver or kidney problems, glaucoma, epilepsy, Parkinson's disease, prostate problems, a small intestinal blockage, porphyria.

Evidence for its use: The authors of Clinical Evidence in 2007 concluded "We found no direct information from RCTs about the effects of cinnarizine in the treatment of people with acute attacks of Ménière's disease." (RCT – randomized, controlled trial)

There are studies comparing cinnarizine to other Ménière's drugs and many personal stories of success and doctors observing patients having improvement while taking the drug. Again, without a large controlled study there is no way to know if this is due to the normal fluctuations of Ménière's disease.

REFERENCES:

http://www.services.medicines.org.uk/emc/medicine/7595, accessed May, 2017.

http://www.drugbank.ca/drugs/DB00568 Accessed Sept 22, 2017

James, A.L.and Thorp, M.A. "Menière's disease." *Clinical Evidence* (Online), Mar 1;2007. pii: 0505.

FLUNARIZINE

Flunarizine is a vestibular symptom blocker, not an anti-Ménière's disease drug. It is effective against acute and chronic vertigo, whether caused by abnormal vestibular function or vascular disorders. This drug is somewhat similar to cinnarizine because it is both a calcium channel blocker and an antihistamine. The calcium channel blocking properties in Flunarizine are stronger than its relative, cinnarizine, and it's not in use for motion sickness. It is prescribed for the vertigo of Ménière's disease and used in migraine, peripheral vascular disease and sometimes for epilepsy.

Other names include: Sibelium, Rizelium.

How it works: As a calcium channel blocker it reduces spasm in blood vessels and as an antihistamine it suppresses the histamine response.

Timing: Reaches it's highest level in the blood stream in 2-4 hours, takes 18 days for half the drug to leave the body. Should be used at least one month to evaluate effectiveness. Can take a month or more for the full affect to be felt.

Side effects: Drowsiness, depression, weight gain, extrapyramidal effects, nausea, heartburn, dry mouth, anxiety, skin rash, depression, tremor, difficulty moving, uncontrolled movements.

Interactions: Alcohol, sedatives, anti-anxiety medications, muscle relaxants, tranquilizers, anti-seizure drugs. Increased chance of extrapyramidal effects when used with other drugs with the same side effect.

Caution, do not use if: Depressed, severely constipated, have Parkinson's disease, liver disease or low blood pressure.

Check with your doctor before using if you have: Liver or kidney problems, glaucoma, epilepsy, Parkinson's disease, prostate problems, a small intestine blockage, porphyria.

Evidence for its use: Somewhat weak, no randomized controlled studies can be found in the medical literature. In 1984 32 patients were monitored while taking the drug. Researchers found: "In the final evaluation, the action of flunarizine was generally considered very beneficial both by the attending physicians and the patients."

REFERENCES:

http://pubchem.ncbi.nlm.nih.gov/summary/summary.cgi?cid=5282407, accessed May 2017.

http://www.drugbank.ca/drugs/DB04841, accessed May 2017.

Haid T. "Evaluation of flunarizine in patients with Menière's disease. Subjective and vestibular findings." *Acta Otolaryngologica Supplement, 460*:149-53, 1988.

James, A.L. and Thorp, M.A. "Menière's disease." *Clinical Evidence* (Online), Mar 1;2007. pii: 0505.

Lepcha, A., Amalanathan, S., Augustine, A.M., Tyagi, A.K. and Balraj, A. "Flunarizine in the prophylaxis of migrainous vertigo: a randomized controlled trial." *European Archives of Otorhinolaryngology, 271*(11):2931-2936, 2013.

Van Nueten, J.M. and Vanhoutte, P.M. *New Drugs Annual: Cardiovascular Drugs,* Vol. 2, edited New York: Raven Press, 1984.

CHAPTER TWENTY-FIVE
STEROIDS

Steroids occur naturally in the body and are crucial for the body's response to stress as well as necessary to use the sugars, fats and electrolytes, human beings need for their survival.

The goal of giving extra steroids in Ménière's disease is to decrease local swelling, decrease inflammation and/or reduce or stop an immune attack on the inner ear, called an autoimmune attack. It's thought that the glucosteroid receptors in the inner ear have a positive effect on blood flow.

INTO THE EAR

Dexamethasone can't be placed directly into the inner ear. Instead it's placed into the middle ear from where it can make its way into the inner ear through the oval and round windows. This procedure is called transtympanic dexamethasone injection or intratympanic dexamethasone.

There are several ways this can be accomplished:
- Injection directly through the eardrum with a small syringe, done in the doctor's office.

- Insertion of an ear tube/grommet through the eardrum and then using steroid ear drops at home.

- Insertion of an ear tube/grommet through the eardrum, placing a wick through it and then using steroid ear drops at home.

This treatment is a bit different because the go to source for evidence based medicine, The Cochrane Database, has found "The results of a single trial provide limited evidence to support the effectiveness of intratympanic steroids in patients with Ménière's disease." This trial demonstrated a statistically and clinically significant improvement of the frequency and severity of vertigo measured 24 months after the treatment was administered." This is how a successful treatment looks at the beginning.

Some study results:
- 56 study members, 22 receiving the steroid once a day for three days had complete vertigo control in 40.9 and substantial in 18.2, 34

receiving it once a week for three weeks with complete control in 44.1, substantial in 14.7.

- 32 members given 3 transtympanic injections of dexamethasone over a two-week period. 47% had improvement of vertigo, 41% had improvement or no change in hearing and 59% had a decrease in tinnitus.

- 22 members studied for 2 years. 11 received dexamethasone transtympanically and 11 received a placebo, saline, transtympanically over 5 days. 9 of the 11 receiving the drug had complete control of their vertigo compared to only 4 of 11 receiving plain saline. Hearing was improved in 35% of steroid users and in only 10% of the others and aural fullness improved in 45% of the steroid users and in 20% of the saline group.

- Phase 1b randomized, double-blind, placebo-controlled clinical study looking at a sustained release version of dexamethasone, Oto-104, with 44 members in three groups, placebo, 3mg dose and 12mg. Results were vertigo control in 42% of placebo group, 56% in the 3mg group and 73% in the 12 mg group.

- Phase 2b randomized, double-blind placebo-controlled, study over 5 months had results showing that the drug should go into phase 3 trials.

The purpose of a phase 1b study is to determine the safety and appropriate dose for a new treatment. The phase 2b looks at safety and how well the dose under study has worked. This drug has more study before it can be approved in the U.S.

The company Otonomy developed OTO-104. They have FDA fast track designation so OTO-104 will be brought to market as fast as possible if it is not found to be harmful and is found to be better than giving a placebo.

The goal of the sustained release dexamethasone is giving a uniform dose over a period of time. This should reduce the number of doctor's visits and number of holes through the tympanic membrane.

One risk is the hole through the tympanic membrane might not seal. This might require treatment, even a minor surgical procedure to fix it. The hole usually seals in 18 days. One study of 192 people undergoing the treatment found 3 people with an unsealed hole. People who have had radiation therapy of the head or neck have a higher risk that their hole will not deal on its own.

How widespread is its use? A 2017 U.S. study found roughly 50% of neurotologists and 10% of otolaryngologists offer this treatment.

BLOODSTREAM

Although being used less frequently steroids can also be placed into the bloodstream by either injection or pill. Once in the bloodstream steroids travel throughout the body to many places an autoimmune attack can occur or originate from.

Several steroids can be used including prednisone, dexamethasone (Decadron) and methylprednisolone. The amount and length of time these are used varies greatly from doctor to doctor. Some give a small amount over one or two weeks while others may prescribe it for weeks, months or even longer.

This treatment is usually not given to people with diabetes mellitus, a history of stomach ulcers, high blood pressure, poor thyroid function, cataracts, Cushing Syndrome, fungus infection, myasthenia gravis, colitis, recent surgery, osteoporosis, tuberculosis, heart disease, liver disease, kidney disease, who are pregnant or breast feeding or have an active herpes simplex infection. The pill form should be taken with milk or food.

When placed into the bloodstream these drugs have an amazing number and variety of side effects including weight gain, abnormal hair growth, insomnia, impaired healing, difficulty fighting infection and many more, particularly if the drug is used for months or years. When used for only a week or two the side effects are more limited. If your doctor is suggesting long-term use of steroids question them very carefully about all the options as well as the potential side effects.

An odd thing happens when steroids are placed into the bloodstream for long periods of time (usually months and longer), the body no longer makes its own steroids in the same amounts, a situation called drug induced secondary adrenocortical insufficiency. If the prescribed steroids are stopped suddenly the body can go into a very serious crisis situation with the potential for serious injury, even death on rare occasion. NEVER, EVER decide on your own to stop taking steroid pills. They must be stopped slowly by reducing the strength of the pill over time, something that should only be done under the direction of a primary care provider with experience in the procedure.

Some doctors may place steroids into the blood stream at the same time dexamethasone is given transtympanically.

If taking steroids long-term get and wear medic alert jewelry available online at www.medicalert.org or via snail mail at MedicAlert Foundation International, 2323 Colorado Avenue, Turlock, CA 95382, 888-633-4298

Insurance consideration: An insurance company may view transtympanic dexamethasone as investigational or unproven for general use. If this treatment has been suggested get insurance company approval before going forward with it.

If current studies go well, and the drug is approved by the FDA in the U.S insurance companies will have more trouble rejecting this treatment.

REFERENCES:

Barrs, D.M., Keyser, J. S., Stallworth, C. and McElveen, J.T. "Intratympanic steroid injections for intractable Ménière's disease." *Laryngoscope, 111*(12): 2100-2104, 2001.

Barrs, D. M. "Intratympanic injections of dexamethasone for long-term control of vertigo." *Laryngoscope, 114(11):*1910-1914, 2004.

Bolease-Aquirre, M.S., Lin, F.R., Della-Santina, C.C., Minor, L.M. and Carey, J.P. "Longitudinal results with intratympanic dexamethasone in the treatment of Ménière's disease." *Otology and Neurotology, 29*(1):33-38, 2008.

Chandrasekhar, S.S., Rubinstein, R.Y., Kwartler, J.A., Gatx, M., Connelly, P.E., Huang, E. and Baredes, S. "Dexamethasone pharmacokinetics in the inner ear: comparison of route of administration and use of facilitating agents." *Otolaryngology-Head & Neck Surgery, 122(4)*:521-528, 2000.

Dodson, K.M., Woodson, E. and Sismanis, A. "Intratympanic steroid perfusion for the treatment of Ménière's disease: a retrospective study." *Ear Nose Throat Journal, J83(6):*394-398, 2004.

Doyle, K.J., Bauch, C., Battista, R., Beatty, C., Hughes, G.B., Mason, J., Maw, J. and Musiek, F.L."Intratympanic steroid treatment: a review." *Otology and Neurotology, 25(6):*1034-1039, 2004.

Farhoos, Z. and Lambert, P.R. "The physiologic role of corticosteroids in Meniere's disease." *American Journal of Otolaryngology, 37*(5):455-458, 2016.

Garduno-Anaya, M.A., De Toledo, H.C., Hinojosa-Gonzalez, R., Pane-Pianese, C. and Rios-Castameda, L.C. "Dexamethasone inner ear perfusion by intratympanic injection in unilateral Ménière's disease: a two-year prospective, placebo-controlled, double-blind, randomized trial." *Otolaryngology-Head and Neck Surgery, 133*(2):285-294, 2005.

Hochadel, M. *The AARP Guide to Pills*. New York: Sterling Publishing Company, Inc., 2005.

Hoffer, M.E., Gottshall, K.R., Balough, B.J. and Wester, D. "Oral and transtympanic steroid treatment in new onset Ménière's disease." Abstract of the 5th Ménière's Disease Meeting, 2005.

Itoh, A. and Sakata, E. "Treatment of vestibular disorders." *Acta Otolaryngologica Suppl, 481*:617-623, 1991.

Lambert, P.R., Nguyen, S., Maxwell, K.S., Tucci, D.L., Lustig, L.R., Fletcher, M., Bear, M. and Lebel C. "A randomized, double-blind, placebo-controlled clinical study to assess safety and clinical activity of OTO-104 given as a single intratympanic injection in patients with unilateral Ménière's disease." *Otology and Neurotology, 33(7)*:1257-1265, 2012.

Lamber, P.R., Carey, J., Mikulec, A.A. and LeBel, C. "Intratympanic sustained-exposure dexamethasone thermosesitive gel for symptoms of Meniere's disease. Randomized phase 2b safety and efficacy trial." *Otology and NEurotology, 37*(10):1669-1676, 2016.

Martin-Sanz, E., Zschaeck, C., Gonzalez, M., Mato, T., Rodrigañez, L., Barona, R. and Sanz. R. "Control of vertigo after intratympanic corticoid therapy for unilateral Ménière's disease: a comparison of weekly versus daily fixed protocols." *Otology and Neurotology, 34*(8):1429-1433, 2013.

Morales-Luckie, E., Cornejo-Suarez, A., Zaragoza-Contreras, M.A. and Gonzalez-Perez, O. "Oral administration of prednisone to control refractory vertigo in Ménière's disease: a pilot study." *Otology and Neurotology, 26*(5):1022-1026, 2005.

Phillips, J.S. and Westerberg, B. "Intratympanic steroids for Ménière's disease or syndrome." *Cochrane Database Systematic Review, 6*(7):CD008514, 2011.

Piu, F., Wang, X., Fernandez, R., Dellamary, L., Harrop, A., Ye, Q., Sweet, J., Tapp, R., Dolan, D.F., Altschuler, R.A., Lichter, J.and LeBel, C. "OTO-104: a sustained-release dexamethasone hydrogel for the treatment of otic disorders." *Otology and Neurotology, 32*(1):171-179, 2011.

Rutt, A.L., Hawkshaw, M.J. and Sataloff, R.T. "Incidence of tympanic membrane perforation after intratympanic steroid treatment through myringotomy tubes." *Ear Nose Throat Journal, 90*(4):E21, 2011.

Silverstein, H., Isaacson J.E., Olds, M.J., Rowan, P.T. and Rosenberg, S. "Dexamethasone inner ear perfusion for the treatment of Ménière's disease: a prospective, randomized, double-blind, crossover trial." *American Journal of Otology, 19(2)*:196-201, 1998.

Topf, M.C., Hsu, D.W., Adams, D.R., Zhan, T, Pelosi, S., Wilcox, T.O. McGettigan, B. and Fisher, K.W. "Rate of tympanic membrane perforation after intratym[anic steroid injection." *American Journal of Otolaryngology, 38*(1):21-25, 2017.

Wang, X., Dellamary, L, Fernandez, R., Harrop, A., Keithley, E.M., Harris, J.P., Ye, Q., Lichter J., LeBel, C. and Piu F. "Dose-Dependent Sustained Release of Dexamethasone in Inner Ear Cochlear Fluids Using a Novel Local Delivery Approach." *Audiology and Neurotology, 14*(6):393-401, 2009.

CHAPTER TWENTY-SIX
ANTIVIRAL DRUGS

Doctors who feel Ménière's disease has a viral cause prescribe antiviral drugs. The selection includes acyclovir, famciclovir and valacyclovir. They are used in the treatment of herpes simplex viral infections, especially cold sores, genital herpes and shingles. Most information about these drugs *are* for those three conditions, not for the inner ear.

ACYCLOVIR
This drug has been around since 1983, has a generic form and is the least expensive of the three antivirals. It was the first anti-viral drug and its developer was awarded the Nobel Prize in medicine for this landmark achievement.

Other names: Zovirax

How it comes: Pill form, injection, liquid by mouth

Effects: It prevents the replication of the virus by working inside its DNA. If the virus cannot replicate it stops spreading in the body. The virus is not killed, it is stopped and remains in the body so further flare-ups are possible. The lowly cold sore that can break out from time to time is one example.

How it is taken: Every 4 hours during the day up to a total of five times each 24 hours.

Timing: Leaves the body somewhat fast therefore is taken more times during the day than other anti-virals.

Possible side effects: Diarrhea, nausea and headache are the most common according the original maker, GlaxoSmithKline. Problems are more common in people with kidney disease/impairment.

Interactions: Should not be taken with the anti-gout drug Probenecid (also called benemid, Probalan).

Not recommended for people with serious disorders of the kidney, lungs. Liver, brain or mind (depression, schizophrenia)

Evidence for its use: The original clinical trials were conducted for its use in herpes infections that can be seen and more easily diagnosed than inner ear problems. The trials were in herpes zoster (shingles), chicken pox, cold sores and genital herpes. There are a few small clinical studies in the literature for its use in Ménière's disease but were not as large or well controlled.

VALACYCLOVIR

This drug has been around since 1995, it has a generic form, and it is more expensive than acyclovir, even the generic form is expensive. It

differs from acyclovir because it is a prodrug, the body must turn valacyclovir into acyclovir inside the body before it can work.

Other names: Valtrex

Effects: It prevents the copying or replication of the virus by working inside its DNA. If the virus cannot replicate it stops spreading in the body. The virus is not killed, it is stopped and remains in the body so further flare-ups are possible. An example of this is the lowly cold sore that can break out from time to time for years.

How it comes: Pill form, can be made into a suspension by a pharmacist.

How it is taken: Usually twice daily

Timing: Stays active in the body longer than acyclovir (which is why it's taken only twice daily).

Possible side effects: Most common reported by the original maker GlaxoSMithKline are headache, nausea and abdominal pain in adults, headaches in children. The most serious side effects usually occur in people with kidney disease and the elderly.

Interactions: Should not be taken with the anti-gout drug Probenecid (also called benemid, Probalan).

Evidence for its use: Clinical trials were conducted for its use in herpes infections that could be diagnosed with certainty including herpes zoster (shingles), chicken pox, cold sores and genital herpes. There are a few small clinical studies in the literature for its use in Ménière's disease that have been somewhat positive.

Not recommended for people with serious disorders of the kidney, lungs. Liver, brain or mind (depression, schizophrenia)

Valacyclovir is much more expensive than acyclovir, an insurance company may not cover its cost. Sometimes acyclovir is used first and if it does not have the desired affect valacyclovir is then used. Acyclovir leaves the body more rapidly so must be taken more often. Both are available in generic forms but even that is pricey.

FAMCICLOVIR
Initial approval for this drug in the US was 1994. There is a generic form. Like valacyclor, it is a prodrug, the body turns it into penciclovir before it is effective.

Other names: Famvir.

Effects: It prevents the replication of the virus by working inside its DNA. If the virus cannot replicate it stops spreading in the body. The virus is not killed, it is stopped and remains in the body so further flare-ups are possible. An example of this is the lowly cold sore that can break out from time to time.

Evidence for its use: Clinical trials were conducted for its use in herpes infections that could be diagnosed with certainty including herpes zoster (shingles), chicken pox, cold sores and genital herpes. In one small Ménière's study 25% of the people receiving the drug had a reduction in vertigo spells compared to 18% who were on the placebo. Some reduction in hearing fluctuation was also found.

Possible Side effects: According to the Novartis drug company, 10% of adults may experience headache and/or nausea

REFERENCES:

http://www.accessdata.fda.gov/drugsatfda_docs/label/2008/020487s014lbl.pdf Accessed May, 2017.

http://www.accessdata.fda.gov/drugsatfda_docs/label/2005/018828s030,020089s019,019909s020lbl.pdf Accessed May, 2017.

https://www.pharma.us.novartis.com/sites/www.pharma.us.novartis.com/files/ Accessed May, 2017.

Derebery, M.J., Fisher, L.M. and Igba, I. "Randomized double-blinded placebo controlled clinical trial of famciclovir for reduction of Ménière's disease symptoms." Otolaryngology-Head and Neck Surgery, 131(6):877-884, 2004.

Gacek, R. "A perspective on recurrent vertigo." ORL, 75:91-107, 2013.

Gacek, R.R. "Recovery of hearing in Meniere's disease after antiviral treatment." American Journal of Otolaryngology, 36(3):315-323, 2015.

CHAPTER TWENTY-SEVEN
PRESSURE AS TREATMENT

For year's people with Ménière's disease described being affected by pressure changes. Flying, traveling through mountains, weather changes and scuba diving were all mentioned as affecting symptoms at times. In the 1970's Swedish researchers started studying the effects of positive pressure in people with Ménière's disease. The Meniett® and to a lesser extent, the P-100®, devices are the end result of that research.

The Meniett® and P-100® are portable medical devices designed to deliver controlled, pulsed, positive pressure into the ear to reduce or stop the symptoms of Ménière's disease. The Meniett® was approved in 1999 by the FDA for use in the USA, by Health Canada in 2001, by the Australian Register of Therapeutic Goods (ARTG) in 2001 and has been available from the NHS in the UK since 2002.

The P-100®, is manufactured and sold by Enttex of Germany. As of 2016 the company has not applied for FDA approval and it's only available from an Internet store. One very small study comparing the P-100® and the Meniett® found no difference in their effectiveness. More information about the P-100® can be found on the Enttex webpage: www.enttex.com

Although the inner ear is encased in the temporal bone it can be affected by air pressure via the membrane covered openings (the oval window and the round window) between it and the middle ear. Pressure can be passed from the middle ear to the inner ear but how a few minutes of a treatment reduces symptoms for hours, days or longer isn't known. Some of the theories include:

- Increased pressure affects chemicals such as mineral corticoids, vasopressin or atrial natriuretic hormone that then reduce the pressure exerted by endolymph.

- Endolymph is pushed out through the endolymphatic duct toward the endolymphatic sac by the increased perilymph pressure.

- Oxygenation is improved due to improved circulation.

Treatment begins in the doctor's office with a minor surgical procedure to insert a pressure equalization tube (also known as a ventilation tube, grommet or simply as an ear tube) through the eardrum. The tube allows pressure to pass into the middle ear without disturbing the eardrum. Having an ear tube in place should not be painful. Ear tubes usually don't have to be removed, they generally fall out on their own a few months down the line.

After the tube is inserted a padded earpiece is painlessly inserted into the external ear canal a few times a day for several minutes, the device turned on and the pulsed pressure sent in. The length of time this treatment is needed (days, weeks, months) differs from case to case. There are reports of success with as little as one treatment.

Because a small surgical procedure is required there is some risk involved but it's slight. An allergic reaction, infection and hemorrhage are all theoretical risks but so far no study has found the Meniett® itself to be harmful. Water must be kept out of the ear canal while the pressure equalization tube is in place and until the hole seals up. At least two conditions could be worsened by use of the Meniett®, perilymph fistula (an inner ear condition) and low-pressure hydrocephalus (a brain condition in which there is too much fluid).

A survey of the American Neurotological Society in 2005 found that less than 10% of physicians responding to the survey were using the Meniett® in their practice. Two years later another study named the Meniett® as the most frequently used treatment when diet change didn't work. A 2017 study found 69.2% of otolaryngologists and neurotologist never use pressure as a treatment.

STUDIES
Small but controlled clinical studies have been done in several countries. Most have shown a significant number of people undergoing Meniett® treatments have a reduction in vertigo and an improvement in their general level of function and well being, at least over the short term. The results for aural fullness, tinnitus and hearing loss have not been as good.

All these studies have been relatively small and have the same difficulties Ménière's disease studies suffer from: Small numbers of participants, not sure beyond a reasonable doubt if all the people in the study have the same disorder, the disorder naturally waxes and wanes over time, most studies lack either a control group or placebo group, most are short-term studies, and there is no objective test to measure successful control of vertigo and other vestibular symptoms. All participants have ear tubes inserted which on their own are used as a treatment in some parts of the world. Also, some studies have been conducted by doctors being paid by Xomed, the makers of the Meniett®, creating a potential conflict of interest.

- Australia, 2005: Looked at 18 people over an average of 18 months. 12 had improvements in vertigo and function and 5 had improvement in hearing. Of the 6 who did not improve 4 had prior ear surgery and two had prior gentamicin.

- Belgium, 2005: Three year study of 12 patients who failed drug therapy and were referred for gentamicin treatment instead underwent 2 months of treatment with the Meniett®. Two dropped out of treatment. In the remaining 10 patients researchers found a decrease in number of attacks but no improvement in how they felt or functioned. Six of the original 12 went on to procedures destroying ear function.

- China, 2007: Six month study of 18 patients. None of these 18 had any ill effects over the following 6 months, the group as a whole had a decrease in vertigo severity and frequency, decrease in sick days and an improvement in function. As a group their EcoG had significant changes, their ENG calorics didn't change and 12 of the 18 had a slight hearing loss at 8 weeks.

- Denmark, 2005: Randomized, multicenter, double-blind, placebo controlled study of 40 patients who had had at least 8 attacks in the prior year and attacks continuing for two months after insertion of the ventilation tube. The self-reported function of the active group was statistically better than the placebo group. Comparison of the number of attacks did not show a statistically significant difference.

- France, 2007: Four month study of 53 patients. None of these 53 had any ill effects; vertigo stopped in 65% and was reduced in 24.5%.

- Netherlands, 2006: Studied vestibular function in 32 patients undergoing treatment with the Meniett®. Found no statistically significant changes in function between testing before, during or after Meniett® treatment.

- Sweden 2000: Randomized, placebo controlled, muticenter study of 56 patients. 31 patients completed two weeks with the Meniett® and

25 completed two weeks with the placebo gadget. The Meniett® group had improvements in amount of vertigo, hearing and the ability to function when compared to those in the placebo group.

1997: Placebo controlled randomized study with 39 participants comparing ECOG results. There was a statistically significant difference in the active group and none in the placebo group.

1982: Study with 5 participants, all had hearing improvement and went into remission during the two-year follow-up period.

1975: Study with 3 participants using a pressure chamber, all three had hearing improvement.

- USA
  2006: Two-year placebo controlled multicenter clinical trial with 58 participants on low-sodium diets using the Meniett® three times a day. 39 (67%) either went into remission or were greatly improved, 14 dropped out of the study to pursue surgery for symptoms that had not improved or had worsened, of the 43 that completed the study 20 went into remission, usually in the first year. Of those who went into remission, 16 did so long term. To summarize: 16 of 58 participants went into long-term remission. This was a two-year study so long term remission was less than two years.

P-100® Studies
- Australia, 2005: Compared the Meniett® and P-100® and concluded they were equally successful.

Not all insurance companies will pay for the Meniett® although Medicare now does pay for rental, on a case-by-case basis. Companies not covering it generally say it's experimental or not clinically proven and only pay for treatment in their Medicare customers, not in their other subscribers.

If an insurance company covers the Meniett® they may only do so if the diagnosis is confirmed by a Ménière's disease specialist who certifies standard medical treatment has failed and the only other treatment option is surgery.

Medtronic, maker of the Meniett® and owned by Xomed, has a

Meniett® webpage, www.meniett.com, with information including a sample medical necessity letter (in the patient forms area) that might help to convince an insurance company to cover the surgery (to insert a tube through the eardrum) and use of the Meniett.

Evidence for Use of the Meniett

Unfortunately the go-to source determining the quality of evidence for treatment, Cochrane, has found: "There is no evidence, from five included studies, to show that positive pressure therapy is effective for the symptoms of Ménière's disease. There is some moderate quality evidence, from two studies, that hearing levels are worse in patients who use this therapy. The positive pressure therapy device itself is minimally invasive. However, in order to use it, a tympanostomy tube (grommet) needs to be inserted, with the associated risks. These include the risks of anesthesia, the general risks of any surgery and the specific risks of otorrhoea and tympanosclerosis associated with the insertion of a tympanostomy tube. Notwithstanding these comments, no complications or adverse effects were noted in any of the included studies."

REFERENCES:

Barbara, M., Consagra, C., Monini, S., Nostro, G., Harguindey, A., Vestri, A. and Filipo, R. "Local pressure protocol, including Meniett, in the treatment of Ménière's disease: short-term results during the active stage." *Acta Otolaryngologica, 121*(8):939-944, 2001.

Boudewyns, A.N., Wuyts, F.L., Hoppenbrouwers, M., Ketelslagers, K., Vanspauwen, R., Forton, G. and Van de Heyning, P.H. "Meniett therapy: rescue treatment in severe drug-resistant Ménière's disease?" *Acta Otolaryngologica, 125*(12):1283-1289, 2005.

Clyde, J.W., Oberman, B.S. and Isildak, H. "Current management practices in Meniere's Disease." *Otology and Neurotology*, 38(6):159-167, 2017.

Densert, B., Densert, O., Arlinger, S., Sass, K. and Odkvist, L. "Immediate effects of middle ear pressure changes on the electrocochleographic recordings in patients with Ménière's disease: a clinical placebo-controlled study." *American Journal of Otology*, 18(6):726-733, 1997.

Densert, B. and Densert, O. "Overpressure in treatment of Meniere's disease." *Laryngoscope, 92*(11):1285-92, 1982.

Densert, O., Ingelstedt, S., Ivarsson, A. and Pedersen, K. "Immediate restoration of basal sensorineural hearing (Mb Meniere) using a pressure chamber." *Acta Otolaryngologica, 80*(1-2):93-100, 1975.

Faict, H. and Bouccara, D. "Middle ear overpressure with Meniett in Ménière disease: indications, results at short and middle terms in 53 cases." *Rev Laryngol Otol Rhinol (Bord), 128*(1-2):33-36, 2007.

Franz, B. and van der Laan, F. "P-100 in the treatment of Ménière's disease: a clinical study." *International Tinnitus Journal, 11*(2):146-149, 2005.

Gates, G.A., Verrall, A., Green, J.D., Tucci, D.L. and Telian, S.A. "Meniett clinical trial: long-term follow-up." *Archives of Otolaryngology-Head and Neck Surgery, 132*(12):1311-1616, 2006.

Gates, G.A. "Treatment of Meniere's disease with the low-pressure pulse generator (Meniett device)." *Expert Review of Medical Devices, 2*(5):533-537, 2005.

Ingelstedt S., Ivarsson A. and Tjernström Ö. "Immediate relief of symptoms during acute attacks of Ménière's disease, using a pressure chamber." *Acta Otolaryngol*ogica, 82(5-6):368-378, 1976.

Kim, H.H., Wiet, R.J. and Battista, R.A. "Trends in the diagnosis and the management of Meniere's disease: results of a survey." *Otolaryngology-Head and Neck Surgery*, 132(5):722-726, 2005.

Liu, F. and Huang, W.N. "Clinical short-term effect of Meniett pulse generator for Meniere disease." *Zhonghua Er Bi Yan Hou Tou Jing Wai Ke Za Zhi, 42*(3):169-172, 2007.

Odkvist, L.M., Arlinger, S., Billermark, E., Densert, B., Lindholm, S. and Wallqvist, J. "Effects of middle ear pressure changes on clinical symptoms in patients with Ménière's disease--a clinical multicentre placebo-controlled study." *Acta Otolaryngologica Supplement, 543*:99-101, 2000.

Peterson, W.M. and Isaacson, J.E. "Current Management of Ménière's Disease in an Only Hearing Ear." *Otology and Neurotology*, 28(5):696-699, 2007.

Rajan, G.P., Din, S. and Atlas, M.D. "Long-term effects of the Meniett device in Ménière's disease: the Western Australian experience." *Journal of Laryngology and Otology, 119(5)*:391-395, 2005.

Stokroos, R., Olvink, M.K., Hendrice, N. and Kingma, H. "Functional outcome of treatment of Ménière's disease with the Meniett pressure generator." *Acta Otolaryngologica, 126(3)*:254-258, 2006.

Syed, M.I., Rutka, J.A., Hendry, J. and Browning, G.G. "Positive pressure therapy for Meniere's syndrome/disease with a Meniett device: a systematic review of randomised controlled trials." *Clinical Otolaryngology, 40(3)*:197-207, 2015.

Thomsen, J., Sass, K., Odkvist, L. and Arlinger, S. "Local overpressure treatment reduces vestibular symptoms in patients with Meniere's disease: a clinical, randomized, multicenter, double-blind, placebo-controlled study." *Otology and Neurotology, 26(1)*:68-73, 2005.

van Sonsbeek, S., Pullens, B. and van Benthem, P.P. "Positive pressure therapy for Ménière's disease or syndrome." *Cochrane Database Systematic Review*, 10;3:CD008419. doi: 10.1002/14651858.CD008419.pub2., 2015.

Younger, R., Longridge, N.S. and Mekjavic, I. "Effect of reduced atmospheric pressure on patients with fluctuating hearing loss due to Ménière's disease." *Journal of Otolaryngology, 13:* 76-82, 1984.

http://www.fda.gov/cdrh/pdf/k991562.pdf   accessed June 2017

http://www.meniett.com accessed June 2017

CHAPTER TWENTY-EIGHT
GENTAMICIN

CAUTION: Because it's effects are destructive and permanent, gentamicin treatments should not be rushed into or used as a first treatment. It causes a permanent loss of at least some vestibular function. The treatment cannot be reversed and it is possible, although not probable, to end up in a worse situation than before treatment. Other less harmful treatments such as diuretics and diet change or betahistine (outside the US) should be tried first.

Gentamicin is used to stop attacks of vertigo by poisoning the inner ear it's injected into. This drug is a member of the aminoglycoside antibiotic family. The first aminoglycoside, streptomycin, was developed in the mid-1940's to treat tuberculosis, the deadliest infectious disease of the time. Soon after the drug went into use, a serious side effect, inner ear poisoning (ototoxicity), with hearing loss and balance function impairment, were noticed.

It didn't take ENT's long to figure out they might use this vestibular poisoning to the advantage of people with Ménière's disease having uncontrollable attacks of violent vertigo. Instead of doing surgery to destroy the inner ear they realized the damaged areas could be destroyed chemically.

Streptomycin was the first drug used to intentionally destroy inner ear balance function. The drug was injected into a large muscle from where it entered the blood stream, travelled to both ears and poisoned them. Attempts to poison one ear alone by injecting streptomycin directly into it failed because it caused massive loss of hearing. Gentamicin was developed as an antibiotic in the 1960's and is the aminoglycoside now used to treat Ménière's disease because it doesn't cause the same degree of hearing loss as streptomycin. A 2005 physician survey found 38% of physicians offered gentamicin treatments when diet and drugs failed.

Gentamicin treatments seem to work best in stopping or reducing spontaneous attacks of violent vertigo. Unsteadiness/imbalance as well as vertigo and nausea from head movement or visual stimulation aren't usually helped unless they occur with the attacks of violent vertigo. There's no evidence gentamicin can improve any of the other diagnostic symptoms, i.e. tinnitus, ear fullness or hearing loss. It has also been suggested as a treatment for Tumarkin's otolithic crisis.

Gentamicin is placed into the middle ear from where it can diffuse into the inner ear, a procedure referred to as either transtympanic or intratympanic administration of gentamicin. It can be done by:

- Injection of gentamicin through the eardrum with a small syringe in an office procedure.

- Minor office surgery in which a tube is inserted through the ear drum, a wick placed through that and then ear drops placed into the ear canal at home as directed.

These procedures have the potential for causing hearing loss and/or permanent balance impairment. They also carry the small risk of an allergic reaction or infection. The second procedure carries the risk of the eardrum hole not closing naturally after the ear tube has fallen out or an infection could occur.

Gentamicin treatment aims to stop the spontaneous attacks of violent vertigo by killing off the bad vestibular hair cells and/or decreasing the amount of endolymph made by the inner ear. The term chemical labyrinthectomy isn't entirely accurate because the aim isn't complete destruction and, unlike a surgical labyrinthectomy, hearing isn't intentionally sacrificed.

The most widely accepted method is to give only enough gentamicin to stop the attacks of vertigo and do this with small amounts given weeks apart. The other way is to give enough to measurably reduce vestibular function. Reduction in function is determined either by vestibular testing or the appearance of imbalance, difficulty walking or constant vertigo. The first method causes fewer cases of hearing loss and imbalance.

One standard number of injections doesn't work for everyone. Dosing of gentamicin is done a bit by trial and error; one standard amount doesn't work for everyone. One study of 57 people receiving gentamicin from the same institution found 49.1% only needed one injection and the rest needed between 2 and 10 spaced as much as 4 weeks apart.

Vertigo returns months or years later in some people necessitating another round of gentamicin. Why? Some of the "bad" hair cells may have only been damaged and symptoms return once they heal. Because gentamicin doesn't stop the progression of Ménière's, the disorder may progress to affect areas not destroyed by the gentamicin and symptoms may reappear. Some hair cell regeneration might also take place leading to the return of symptoms.

Hearing loss is possible from the use of gentamicin. In general the larger the dose of gentamicin the higher the risk of hearing loss and the shorter the time between doses the greater the risk to hearing. In other words if gentamicin is given in one big dose once or twice a day everyday for several days the chance of hearing loss is very high compared to one low dose every few weeks.

Because no large studies comparing the use of gentamicin to doing nothing have been done we don't know if a change in hearing after gentamicin is due to the gentamicin or the normal progression of the Ménière's disease.

After treatment with gentamicin most people hardly miss a day of work while others have problems and may need vestibular rehabilitation to get back to full speed. It's unknown what percentage has ear fullness and/or tinnitus change.

The symptoms of vestibular destruction range from none all the way to vertigo and vomiting for days. What a person will experience depends upon:

- How much vestibular function was left in the ear when the treatment begins.
- The amount of destruction done by the treatment.
- How rapidly the damage occurs.

The strongest symptoms come from rapid, massive damage in an ear that had lots of good vestibular function left. This is not likely when gentamicin injections are low dose and given weeks apart.

Possible adverse effects: Allergy, irritation, eardrum perforation, hearing loss, lose of too much balance function.

EVIDENCE FOR ITS USE
Studies claim success in 75 to 95% of patients. Some consider complete control of vertigo attacks as success and others consider "good" control to be success.

In 2015 a group of physicians looking at all studies of gentamicin concluded gentamicin works on vertigo in many people. They also found no consensus on the dose to use or treatment protocol to follow.

No studies look at what happens if the second ear goes on to develop Ménière's. We do know that some people have a return of symptoms and are successfully treated with more gentamicin.

Options, if the gentamicin treatment is ineffective, include doing nothing, more gentamicin, trying physical therapy, Meniett endolymphatic sac surgery or destructive surgery.

REFERENCES:

Bertino, G., Durso, D., Manfrin, M., Casati, L. and Mira, E. "Intratympanic gentamicin in monolateral Meniere's disease: our experience." *European Archives of Otorhinolaryngology, 263*(3):271-275, 2006.

Bodmer, D., Morong, S., Stewart, C., Alexander, A., Chen, J.M. and Nedzelski, J.M. "Long-term vertigo control in patients after intratympanic gentamicin instillation for Ménière's disease." *Otology and Neurotology, 28*(8):1140-1144, 2007.

Boleas-Aguirre, M.S., Sánchez-Ferrandiz, N., Guillén-Grima, F. and Perez, N. "Long-term disability of class A patients with Ménière's disease after treatment with intratympanic gentamicin." *Laryngoscope, 117*(8):1474-1481, 2007.

Chia, S.H., Gamst, A.C., Anderson, J.P. and Harris, J.P. "Intratympanic gentamicin therapy for Ménière's disease: a meta-analysis." *Otology and Neurotology, 25*(4):544-552, 2004.

Cohen-Kerem, R., Kisilevsky, V., Elinarson, T.R., Kozer, E., Koren, G. and Rutka, J.A. "Intratympanic gentamicin for Meniere's disease: a meta-analysis." *Laryngoscope, 114*(12):2085-2091, 2004.

Colletti, V., Carner, M. and Colletti, L. "Auditory results after vestibular nerve section and intratympanic gentamicin for Ménière's disease." *Otology and Neurotology, 28*(2):145-151, 2007.

De Beer, L., Stokroos, R. and Kingma, H. "Intratympanic gentamicin therapy for intractable Ménière's disease." *Acta Otolaryngologica, 127*(6):605-612, 2007.

Diamond, C., O'Connell, D.A., Hornig, J.D. and Liu, R. "Systematic review of intratympanic gentamicin in Meniere's disease." *Journal of Otolaryngology, 32*(6):351-361, 2003.

Flanagan, S., Mukherjee, P. and Tonkin, J. "Outcomes in the use of intratympanic gentamicin in the treatment of Ménière's disease." *Journal of Laryngology and Otology, 120*(2):98-102, 2006.

Kim, H.H., Wiet, R.J. and Battista, R.A. "Trends in the diagnosis and the management of Meniere's disease: Results of a survey." *Otolaryngology-Head and Neck Surgery, 132*(5):722-726, 2005.

Marzo, S.J. and Leonetti, J.P. "Intratympanic gentamicin therapy for persistent vertigo after endolymphatic sac surgery." *Otolarygology-Head and Neck Surgery, 126*(1):31-33, 2002.

Minor, L.B. "Intratympanic gentamicin for control of vertgio in Meniere's disease: vestibular signs that specify completion of therapy." *American Journal of Otology, 20*(2):209-219, 1999.

Obholzer, R.J. and Wareing, M.J. "Intratympanic gentamicin for Ménière's disease; a survey of current UK practice." *Journal of Laryngology and Otology, 117*:459-461, 2008.

Pullens, B and van Benthem, P.P. "Intratympanic gentamicin for Ménière's disease or syndrome." Cochrane Database Sytematic Review. 2011 Mar 16 CD0088234 doi: 10.1002/14651858.CD

Salt, A.N., Gill, R.M. and Plontke, S.K. "Dependence of Hearing Changes on the Dose of Intratympanically-Applied Gentamicin: A Meta-analysis using Mathematical Simulations of Clinical Drug Delivery Protocols." *Laryngoscope*, *118*(10):1793–1800, 2008.

Syed, M.I., Ilan, O., Nassas, J. and Rutka, J.A. "Intratympanic therapy in Meniere's syndrome or disease up to date evidence of clinical practice." *Clinical Otolaryngology*, *40*(6):682-690, 2015.

Viana, L.M., Bahmad. F. and Rauch, S.D. "Intratympanic gentamicin as a treatment for drop attacks in patients with Meniere's disease." *Laryngoscope*, *124*(9):2151-2154, 2014.

Watson, G.J., Nelson, C. and Irving, R.M. "Is low-dose intratympanic gentamicin an effective treatment for Ménière's disease: the Birmingham experience." *Journal of Laryngology and Otology*, 129(10):970-973, 2015.

Wu, I.C. and Minor, L.B. "Long-term hearing outcome in patients receiving intratympanic gentamicin for Ménière's disease." *Laryngoscope, 113*(5):815-820. 2003.

CHAPTER TWENTY-NINE
SURGERY

No surgery has been scientifically shown to cure, reverse the damage or stop the progression of Ménière's disease. Despite this, surgery may be offered and can be the right treatment for some people.

Surgery for Ménière's disease ranges from a simple ear tube (most common in Europe) to complete destruction of the inner ear. It is usually reserved for cases when nothing less drastic has helped and the symptoms can't be lived with.

THE DECISION

Surgery is never a quick fix or a sure thing; it's just one more treatment option, with more risk, to consider. It should never be rushed into. If you have tried a number of medical treatments without any luck and if your vestibular symptoms are intolerable surgery might be the best choice.

Should surgery be done? This question can only be answered by the person considering the surgery, they alone know how much they're suffering, and how their life has been affected and how many medical treatments they've tried.

DO NOT have surgery if you don't trust your doctor, if you don't understand what you're getting into, if you don't understand the possible benefits of the surgery along with the risks or if your questions haven't been answered satisfactorily. Never consider it because, "things can't get much worse." They can.

Questions your doctor should answer:
- Are you sure the problem is coming from the inner ear? How sure?
- Is the other ear OK?
- Are you sure surgery will help? How sure?
- Can something else be done instead of surgery?
- What are all the risks of the surgery and anesthesia?
- How many of these surgeries have you done?
- How many were successes?
- What do you consider success?
- How many people were made worse? In what way?

- What percent had complications and what were they? (Terms like rare or unlikely aren't good enough, try and get some numbers)

- What will you do for me if the surgery doesn't work or makes me worse?

Ask for the statistics for their patients, not statistics published by another surgeon. Make sure all your questions are answered, the answers can be understood and seem logical. It might help to take someone along to the doctors' office for moral support and to help listen to the doctor.

Making a decision like this is difficult. Take the time and energy to do it right. Clear your schedule and your mind and really think it through. Don't rush into surgery. Look into your soul too. If you have surgery and a bad result can you live with it? - or - Can you live with it if you don't make the effort to have surgery?

GENERAL RISKS OF SURGERY

All surgery has risk involved. How much risk depends upon which surgery is being considered, the health of the person having the surgery, the type of anesthesia used and the health care professionals doing it.

Some people are more at risk from surgery than others. Folks with serious disorders such as diabetes, heart disease, respiratory disease, history of having had a brain attack (stroke), undergoing treatment for blood clotting (particularly with a drug such as Coumadin), liver disease, kidney disease or a system wide autoimmune disorder are at the highest risk. A specialist needs to know if a person has a serious illness or difficulties with healing, infection or bleeding, in addition to their vestibular disorder. Surgery should also be discussed with the PCP and other specialists being seen.

Every surgery has the risk of infection, excessive bleeding, or having the wrong thing cut or damaged. When something does go badly it usually affects hearing, balance, taste, or facial nerve function. Each surgery described later includes more information about risk.

General anesthesia has some risk as well because multiple, potent drugs that circulate rapidly throughout the body may be used. On occasion people have allergic or other bad reactions to these drugs, and very, very rarely can die from a reaction.

In addition to drugs, a breathing tube is inserted during general anesthesia that frequently causes a sore throat and on very rare occasion a fat lip or broken tooth.

BALANCE RISKS
Surgery, at times, can lead to increased vestibular symptoms and/or decreased balance ability.

After surgery designed to stop balance signals from arriving in the brain there will be a period of severe symptoms followed by a recuperation period and a return to normal (if the other ear is normal and the brain able to chemically compensate).

The risk of this surgery is that the other ear really isn't normal and/or the brain can't chemically compensate for the change. If either is the case a person can be left with increased symptoms and a lot of difficulty moving around, particularly in the dark or on an angled surface.

A further risk is that the surgery will go well but the opposite ear will start having problems at a later time leaving a person with less balance function than if they had not undergone the surgery. If this happens there may also be more visual difficulties, possibly even bouncing vision (oscillopsia).

THE SURGERIES
Surgeries for vestibular symptoms aren't all done on the inner ear. They sometimes are also done on surrounding areas like the eardrum, middle ear, and mastoid bone.

Eardrum
Insertion of an ear tube (tympanostomy)
A tube with one end in the external ear canal and one end in the middle ear is inserted during this surgery. Adults usually have it done in the doctor's office using local anesthesia. Children usually require general anesthesia.

Local anesthesia is given, a hole is made through the eardrum with a scalpel or LASER and a very small, short tube inserted. The tube is not stitched in place and most tubes will fall out months down the road. There are several models of tubes in use with some tubes staying in place longer then others.

Tubes come in a number of sizes and shapes. The T-shaped model can stay in place indefinitely while the others fall out over weeks to months.

This surgery isn't done very often for vestibular problems in the US. When it is, there are four reasons it might be done:

- To place medication into the middle ear from where it can travel to the inner ear.
- As the first step in using a pressure machine for treatment of Ménière's disease.
- To allow equal air pressure on both sides of the eardrum.
- To limit movement of the eardrum.

Because this surgery is usually done with local anesthesia it is low risk surgery. The most common problem occurring is a failure of the hole to close up once the tube is out. This occurs more frequently with the T-shaped models. Treatment for this is a patch. Infections also occur on occasion.

After an ear tube insertion most people go immediately back to their usual activities with restrictions on getting water into the ear canal while swimming and similar activities.

In Europe placement of a tube is sometimes done as a treatment for the vertigo of Ménière's disease. There is no good explanation of why this would decrease vertigo but at least one little study found improvement in some people having it done.

Inner Ear

All these surgeries begin with a mastoidectomy.

Mastoidectomy

A mastoidectomy is a partial removal of the bone behind the ear called the mastoid bone. Some hair must be shaved from the area behind the ear, and a C-shaped incision is done that may require stitches and will leave a scar.

Depending upon how the surgery is done a depression may be left behind the ear that interferes a bit with wearing glasses in some people. This area may also be sensitive to touch and pressure for months or more after the surgery. A procedure requiring more time and skill can be done toavoid a large depression – ask your surgeon about this if it's a concern.

No matter why a mastoidectomy is done there are some common problems possible after it. Fluid may collect in the middle ear and cause reduced hearing for several days. Areas of numbness may occur on, and behind, the external ear that usually improves over time. The sense of taste may be temporarily disrupted. The end of the eustachian tube may be swollen shut causing sound distortion and possibly some pain, particularly while swallowing. Unexpected problems can occur as well including infection, hearing loss, disturbed vestibular function, increased tinnitus and facial nerve damage.

Endolymphatic Sac Surgeries
This is the most controversial Ménière's disease surgery. It is the only one that has been studied with a placebo group. A number of people with Ménière's disease consented to a study where half had the real surgery and half only had the preliminary mastoidectomy. The results of the surgery were then studied and no difference found between the two groups. Despite this some doctors feel there is a place for its use.

Another study looked at the temporal bones of 15 people who had endolymphatic sac surgery and found only 2 people had the shunt properly placed as intended. Despite this 8 of the 15 people did have relief from vertigo. The two with the shunt properly placed did not have relief from vertigo. Researchers concluded: "Endolymphatic sac surgery does not relieve hydrops in patients with Ménière's syndrome. Yet, sac surgery relieves vertigo in some patients, but the mechanism of such symptomatic relief remains unknown."

Another review of results concluded: "ESS is a surgical option for MD that offers relief from vertigo in selected patients, but patients need to be cautioned about the risk of hearing loss and the requirement for subsequent destructive treatment in a significant proportion of cases."

They found only 35% of patients with complete vertigo control and 33% with deteriorating hearing after the surgery.

There are a number of surgeries in this category including endolymphatic sac decompression, endolymphatic sac shunt and endolymphatic sac valve insertion. They are all done in an attempt to control the amount of endolymph in the inner ear. All begin with a mastoidectomy and are followed by removal of bone until the endolymphatic sac can be found.

- Decompression: The endolymphatic sac is located and bone around it removed. It's believed this will improve circulation to the sac or allow it to expand so it can work better or hold more endolymphatic fluid.

- Shunt: The endolymphatic sac is found, an opening made into it and either a premade straw-like tube or a piece of silastic sheeting inserted with the other end left in the mastoid space. In the past a small hole was made through the skull into the space around the brain where the end of the tube was placed.

- Valve: In this version of the surgery a manufactured pressure release valve is implanted instead of the straw or sheeting. The idea here is that excess endolymphatic fluid will escape only as needed.

All of these procedures are done with general anesthesia as "same day surgery" which means showing up at the surgical center in the morning and leaving in the afternoon or early evening. The amount of pain experienced is usually minimal and most people can resume normal activities a day or two after the surgery. Instructions usually include not shampooing the hair for a number of days.

In addition to the chance of failure, this type surgery can also cause hearing loss (possibly even deafness), infection, serous labyrinthitis, persistent spinal fluid leak, an increase in vestibular symptoms, or facial nerve damage. According to published reports this surgery causes hearing loss or deafness in 5% of people.

Some surgeons perform these surgeries regularly and others never do them because they feel after a year or two people who have had the surgery are no better off than those who have not had it.

The success rates of published reports vary from 50 to 75%. A reduction in symptoms may not be immediate and might take several weeks. One study comparing the Meniett, gentamicin and endolymphatic shunt found "no differences were found between the three treatment options in terms of patients going on to definitive labyrinthectomy or in the number of months of symptom relief following treatment."

Labyrinthectomy
This surgery is done to stop attacks of violent vertigo in people who have lost all, or nearly all, hearing in the ear.

There are two general ways it can be done; with an incision behind the ear (i.e. after first doing a mastoidectomy) or through the middle ear (after first doing a tympanotomy). The first surgery is called the transmastoid approach and the second the transcanal approach. Sometimes a third version is done, the translabyrinthine vestibular nerve section.

- Transmastoid approach: All five balance parts of the inner ear; the contents inside the ampulla of the posterior, horizontal, and anterior semicircular canals and the maccula of the utricle and saccule, are removed. This is done by drilling through the temporal bone to each of the five spots and scraping or sucking out the cells in these microscopic areas.

- Transcanal labyrinthectomy: A tympanotomy is done, the oval window pierced and a vacuum like device used to suck out the contents of the inner ear.

- Translabyrinthine vestibular nerve section: After removing all five balance areas further surgery is done to cut the vestibular nerve within the internal auditory canal.

Hearing is lost due to the trauma of the surgery in all three versions of this surgery.

Following surgery, symptoms range from nothing more than a bit of pain when lifting the head up off the bed to horrific vertigo and vomiting for days that must be treated with drugs. People missing the most vestibular function before surgery have the least amount of vestibular symptoms after the surgery and those with the most vestibular function left, at the time of the surgery, have the most symptoms.

Sometimes vestibular rehabilitation therapy begins the day after surgery to help the brain chemically compensate. Recuperation to the point of returning to work and "normal" activities varies, a lot. It can take a week for some people and several months for others. For a few people this may never be complete.

The risks of this surgery include facial nerve damage that could cause permanent drooping of the face and eyelid on one side of the face, an increase in tinnitus, persistent spinal fluid leak, infection, hematoma or collection of blood, taste disturbance, and dry mouth.

Also, the vertigo might not be eliminated and/or the brain may not compensate for the total loss of balance function on the one side.

Vestibular nerve section

In this surgery the vestibular branch of the vestibulocochlear nerve is cut to stop the flow of balance information from the ear to the brain. The problem causing the violent attacks of spontaneous vertigo is not fixed, instead the message is prevented from reaching the brain.

It's usually done in people who still have some hearing in the problem ear. If nearly all hearing is gone a labyrinthectomy is more commonly done.

This is one of the more serious vestibular surgeries because the nerve is cut very near the brain. Despite this, the surgery is relatively safe. The hearing and facial nerves are more at risk than the brain in this surgery. The most likely complication from the surgery is further loss of hearing. Other possibilities include facial nerve damage and spinal fluid leak. This usually requires some time in the hospital.

There are several versions of this surgery including: the retrolabyrinthine, middle fossa, retrosigmoid, suboccipital and the combination retrolabyrinthine/retrosigmoid. Most of these begin with a mastoidectomy followed by further drilling until the vestibulocochlear nerve is found in the space near the brain. Many times the empty space left by this surgery is filled in with fat and other tissue from a person's own abdomen or the area behind the ear.

Following the surgery, symptoms range from nothing more than feeling a bit feverish and having some pain when lifting the head up off the pillow to horrific vertigo and vomiting lasting for days. People missing the most vestibular function before surgery have the least amount of vestibular symptoms after the surgery and those with the most vestibular function left at the time of the surgery have the most symptoms.

Cutting the nerve carrying balance information sounds pretty straight forward but is not. The hearing and balance nerve travel part of the way to the brain within the same covering and it is not always possible to find all the vestibular parts. This surgery does not always eliminate the vertigo, possibly because the nerve hasn't been fully cut.

Since transtympanic gentamicin came onto the scene the number of vestibular nerve sections done has dropped significantly.

REFERENCES:

Arenberg, I. K., and Graham, M. *Treatment options for Ménière's Disease: endolymphatic sac surgery: do it or don't do it and why.* San Diego, CA, Singular Publishing Group, 1998.

Basura, G.J., Lin, G.C. and Telian, S.A. "Comparison of Second-Echelon Treatments for Ménière's Disease." *JAMA Otolaryngology- Head and Neck Surgery, 140*(8):754-761, 2014.

Brackmann, D. E., Shelton, C., and Arriaga, M. A. *Otologic surgery.* 4th ed. Philadelphisa Elsevier, 2016.

Bretlau, P., Thomsen, J., Tos, M. and Johnsen, N.J. "Placebo effect in surgery for Meniere's disease. A double-blind placebo-controlled study on endolymphatic sac shunt surgery." *Advances in Otorhinolaryngology, 28*:139-146, 1982.

Bretlau, P., Thomsen, J., Tos, M. and Johnsen, N.J. "Placebo effect in surgery for Meniere's disease: a three-year follow-up study of patients in a double blind placebo controlled study on endolymphatic sac shunt surgery." *American Journal of Otology, 5*(6):558-561, 1984.

Bretlau, P., Thomsen, J., Tos, M. and Johnsen, N.J. "Placebo effect in surgery for Meniere's disease: nine-year follow-up." *American Journal of Otology, 10*(4):259-261, 1989.

Chung, J.W., Fayad, J., Linthicum, F., Ishiyama, A. and Merchant, S.N. "Histopathology after Endolymphatic sac surgery for Meniere's Syndrome." *Otology and Neurotology, 32*(4):660–664, 2011.

Ghossaini, S.N. and Wazen, J.J. "An update on the surgical treatment of Ménière's disease." *Journal of the American Academy of Audiology, 17*:38-44, 2006.

Hu, A. and Parnes, L.S. "10-year review of endolymphatic sac surgery for intractable meniere disease." *Journal of Otolaryngology-Head and Neck Surgery, 39*(4):415-421, 2010.

Kerr, A. G. "Emotional investments in surgical decision making." *Journal of Laryngology and Otology,* 116:575-579, 2002.

Nadol, J. B., and Schuknecht, H.F. *Surgery of the ear and temporal bone.* New York: Raven Press, 1992.

Ogawa, Y., Otsuka, K., Hagiwasa, A., Inagaki, A., Shimizu, S., Nagai, N., Itani, S., Saito, Y. and Suzuki, M. "Clinical study of tympanostomy tube placement for patients with intractable Ménière's disease." *Journal of Laryngology & Otology, 129*:120-125, 2015.

Pullens, B., Giard, J.L., Verschuur, H.P. and van Benthem. P.P. "Surgery for Ménière's disease." *Cochrane Database Systematic Review,* 20;(1):CD005395, 2010.

Rasmussen, A.T. "Studies of the VIIIth cranial nerve of man." Laryngoscope, 50:57-83, 1940.

Reid, C.B., Eisenberg, R., Halmagyi, G.M., and Fagan, P.A. "The outcome of vestibular nerve section for intractable vertigo: the patient's point of view." *Laryngoscope,* 106:1553-1556, 1996.

Silverstein, H. "Use of a new device, the MicroWick, to deliver medication to the inner ear." *Ear Nose Throat Journal,* 78(8):595-598, 600, 1999.

Sood, A.J., Lambert, P.R., Nguyen, S.A. and Meyer, T.A. "Endolymphatic sac surgery for Ménière's disease: a systematic review and meta-analysis." *Otology and Neurotology, 35*(6):1033-1045, 2014.

Teufert, K.B. and Doherty, J. "Endolymphatic sac shunt, labyrinthectomy, & vestibular nerve section in Ménière's disease." *Otolaryngological Clinics of North America, 43*:1091-1111, 2010.

Thomsen, J., Bretlau, P., Tos, M. and Johnsen, N.J. "Meniere's disease: a 3-year follow-up of patients in a double-blind placebo-controlled study on endolymphatic sac shunt surgery." *Advances in Otorhinolaryngology, 30*: 350-354, 1983.

CHAPTER THIRTY
COPING AND STAYING SAFE

Ménière's disease can have a major impact on both the person with it and those around them. "Living on" with Ménière's disease can be a major, daunting task. Most people develop their own ways to make their lives livable and safe. This chapter brings together many ideas to help with life.

Even if you are under a doctor's care they can't be at your side to micromanage your life. You will have to constantly assess your own situation and abilities, symptoms, wants and needs. When to carry on normally and when to stay put are up to you.

GENERAL HEALTH AND WELL-BEING
- Exercise daily by walking and moving your head, arms and legs. More vigorous exercise is even better if you are able to do safely.

- Abstain from alcohol and any other drugs (Valium, Xanax, Dramamine, Antivert, antivomiting drugs) that affect brain function.

- Get enough rest and sleep.

- Eat a healthy diet with fresh fruits and vegetables, limit processed foods.

- Understand what is happening, as well as why, before taking any action or making any big changes.

- Share literature and information with family and friends so they can understand Ménière's is not curable and as many as 1/3 of people with it get no better with routine treatment.

- To undercut the fear of embarrassment in front of other people, educate them about Ménière's disease.

- Get counseling if mentally tormented by the Ménière's or unable to think of anything else.

- When hearing loss interferes with life, hearing amplification and/or learning lip reading may help.

- If feeling that Ménière's is a punishment from God discuss this with your clergyman.

Preparation can be the key to both comfort and safety when dealing with Ménière's disease and all of its issues.

PREPARING FOR AN ATTACK

Have medications and supplies prepared ahead of time and accessible next to your bed, in the car, at work or other places you spend time. Your supplies should include an unused garbage bag, bottle of water, breath mints, moist wipes, and a bell or boat horn as well as a sleeping bag in your car if you live in a location that can get cold and a camping pillow. (An emergency silver heat sheet can be used as well and does not use much storage space)

Have children? Do you want them to see you sick or shield them from this? Decide now and not as an attack is leveling you. Whatever your decision, try to be consistent with other child rearing decisions you've made. Put together a plan for taking care of them when an attack interferes with the normal routine. If you have the responsibility of picking them up at school have a back-up plan. Have a plan to get them fed and taken care of during attacks at home. Perhaps the father or a friend can take them during an attack. Taking care of a spouse or parent? Have plans for this in place as well.

Are you on your own? Mobile communications can be crucial. If you don't have a cell (mobile) phone get one and carry it so you can call for assistance when you need it, even at home or work. Make plans with friends, relatives and neighbors for coming to get you if away from home or to come over and help out a bit if at home.

In the U.S. there are some pay-as-you-go plans that can keep the phone expenses down. Tracphone is one of the best known. AARP has discounts through Consumer Cellular; Jitterbug, as well as Republic Wireless are a few with attractively priced plans.

AFTER AN ATTACK

After an attack safety should be your first concern. Assess your situation and abilities. Don't just sit up, jump off the bed and resume the day without some thought. Sleep for a while if you are fatigued and sleepy. Once you can, sit up, move your head around, move your eyes and then try to get up if you need to get to the bathroom or another location. Once you have your wits about you move your head as freely as possible, don't keep it stiff.

If drugs were taken before or during the attack stay in bed or on the couch for a while until they wear off a bit. Stop taking anti-symptom drugs such Valium, Xanax, Dramamine, Antivert, etc. as soon as possible after an attack.

If unsteady, hold something or someone when trying to move.

Do not drive while still under the effects of any drugs you took or if unbalanced and/or having difficulty with your vision.

In the time between attacks try to get back to your normal activities as soon as you safely can. Comfort is important but not as important as safety.

Physical therapy can't do anything for the attacks of Ménière's themselves but can make the time between attacks more tolerable. A physical therapist educated and experienced in vestibular problems can set up a schedule of exercises designed to get you back on track as fast as possible after an attack. They can make sure you aren't over depending upon some senses more than others, a situation that can lead to very unpleasant symptoms.

In the time between attacks try to get back to your normal activities as soon as you safely can. Comfort is important but not as important as safety.

SAFETY MEASURES TO CONSIDER AROUND THE HOUSE
- Remove small rugs that slide or have corners that could roll up and trip you.

- Install night-lights from bedroom to bathroom.

- Have good lighting by steps and stairs, inside and out.

- Have a flashlight at your side for use in power failures or unlit areas.

- A lightweight head mounted flashlight can allow arm use while walking in the dark.

SHOWER/BATH
- Feel unsteady with your eyes closed? Touching the shower wall with as little as a finger can improve balance.

- Add a shower chair/bench in the short term along with a showerhead extension.

- Steady yourself with hands on the wall while lifting your leg to get into the tub or sit on the edge and put each leg into the tub, one at a time.

- Use a shower mat to prevent slipping.

- Don't step into a wet tub – turn the water on once you have gotten in.

SEEING YOUR FEET

People with reduced balance ability are usually further impaired if they can't see their feet while moving around, in water and going up and down stairs. Bifocals and/or progressive lenses may impair the ability to see the feet as well as carrying things that limit this ability. You might be steadier not using bifocals or progressive lenses while walking, particularly on stairs. Touching a banister with your hand can help with stairs. Don't carry things that take away your ability to see your feet while out and about.

ON ICE AND SLIPPERY SURFACES

- Stand up very straight when walking on snow/ice, don't lean forward while walking unless going uphill.

- Take small steps and if the ground is particularly slippery your feet should not leave the surface, they should be slid along.

- Ski poles can be useful if the tips will dig into the surface.

- Wear shoes/boots that allow normal ankle movement – a good pair of leather hiking boots will do this. Gaiters can be worn to keep snow out of low boots. Big snow boots like Sorel Caribous might restrict ankle movement too much.

- Several companies sell products designed to decrease sliding on ice and packed snow, Yaktrax and Stabilicers are two good products.

- It's best to walk on snow that hasn't been packed down and frozen over.

- Wear a ski helmet if you absolutely must go out in icy conditions such as after an ice storm.

- Roughen the surface of ice or snow with ice chipper or other tool, spread gravel, dirt, even kitty litter on a slippery surface. An ice-melting product can help reduce your risk.

SPORTS
Athletes: Don't throw yourself back into your usual activities without testing your abilities a bit more than usual.

Bicyclists: Your balance getting on and off the bike could be more impaired than riding the bike down the road. Practice mounting and dismounting the bicycle with your helmet on before heading off for a ride. If mounting/dismounting proves to be a long-term problem consider one of the newer models of bicycles with a step threw frame. Always wear a helmet, cycling gloves and eye protection.

Downhill Skiers: Go down the bunny slope first to assess your ability. Always wear a helmet and use poles.

Snowboarders: You may have trouble because you can't use leg movement for quick balance adjustments. If this is a long-term problem consider alpine skiing.
Cross-country skiers: Don't throw yourself down a long slope before testing your abilities a bit. You may need to ski with your legs further apart and consider switching to the skating style which would allow you to make more balance adjustments while moving forward.

Runners: You might notice bouncing vision once you return to running. Simply continuing on a program of running may decrease the bouncing vision. If the bouncing does not decrease over time physical therapy may help.

STRESS
- Learn about and understand as much as you can about this disease.

- When anxious convince yourself you aren't dying and will be OK.

- Learn relaxation techniques to relax your mind and body.

- Tell your friends and colleagues about your disease to be rid of the stress of keeping it hidden or secret.

- Exercise daily, vigorous exercise such as jumping rope or fast walking can recycle the chemicals released during the stress. If this isn't possible find something, perhaps a stationary bicycle.

- Schedule down time daily.

- Get counseling - talk about your thoughts and feelings with a professional.

- If ongoing panic and anxiety are limiting your ability to function, talk to your MD about the possibility of medication. This talk can also be with your primary health care provider.

- Communicate with other people who have Ménière's disease.

THOUGHT AND MEMORY PROBLEMS
Of course removing the cause of the thought and memory problem would be best, but isn't always possible. When not possible some lifestyle changes can help.

General changes:
- Thought and memory problems can be made worse by lack of sleep, fatigue, drugs and alcohol.

- Rest up well before a big or important event.

- Take breaks during a big event – get away from the sound and visual excitement. Even sitting down in a restroom or parked car for a while can help.

- If too drained and sick to work, you're probably too impaired to drive a car.

Memory:
- Carry a notepad in pocket or purse along with a pen or pencil.

- Make or add to a list immediately while thinking about it, don't wait.

- Memorization and other learning should be done in small doses. Study for several minutes at a time many times throughout the day for days to weeks to learn something.

- Students: Don't even think about cramming or pulling an all-nighter for a test – study in advance and get a full night's sleep before a test.

Thought
- Don't make important decisions when taking drugs that slow you down like anti-dizziness and anti-nausea drugs.

- Make big decisions when well rested and symptoms are as mild as possible or gone.

- If having trouble thinking and speaking, take care of important tasks in writing via email or snail mail rather than over the phone.

- If decision-making is difficult find a systematic way to go about it. This can be learned from books and courses or passed along through mentoring.

- Be in the easiest environment where you are at your best when doing important thinking. Sitting in a comfortable chair with your head supported, or even laying down may help.

VISION AND EYE HEALTH
- Yearly eye checks, update glasses when needed.

- If wearing glasses for both distance and close up, evaluate if progressives, trifocals or bifocals are a problem, switch to separate reading, distance and computer glasses for the separate activities as need be.

- Wear sunglasses outside to cut down on glare, a baseball cap will cut down some glare as well.

- Exercises as prescribed by a physician or physical therapist should be done as instructed, don't hold back but don't overdo them either.

- If glare is an issue don't drive at night.

- Use a shopping cart in supermarkets and shops for added stability.

- Read in a visually quiet place.

- Place a ruler or other straight edged object under the line of print to help with reading.

- Read in natural light.

- Read sitting down or with the head supported.

THE NECK

Do not use a neck brace to hold your head steady unless your physician has instructed you to do so. It obstructs the view of your feet and the ground, impedes compensation after an attack and may worsen or prolong the very symptoms you are trying to avoid.

DRIVING

Laws regulating driving differ between countries and in the U.S. they differ between states. One goal they all have in common is safety. None want impaired people behind the wheel.

Both distracted and drunk driving causes accidents out on the roads. The symptoms of Ménière's' disease can be a huge distraction as they reduce your ability to react fast enough to changes on the road. Driving while influenced by drugs such as Dramamine, Valium and Xanax is just as dangerous.

If you are told to stop driving, stop. This is not a punishment; it aims to keep you and people around you safe.

SECTION V
RESEARCH

CHAPTER THIRTY-ONE
HISTORY OF RESEARCH

At its very beginning the practice of medicine relied upon observations made by individual physicians as well as beliefs held by their particular society. What they were taught and what they personally witnessed formed the basis of their practice. Substances such as "bad bile," which we now know never existed, were blamed for diseases. Religious beliefs and divine retribution were accepted as the cause of disease in a person who might deserve it.

There was no scientific method to follow, so no real research. No precise way to gather together information from many people. For most of history the profession of medicine knew little about what was inside the human body or how it worked.

Up until the last few decades medicine relied more upon observations by individual doctors and not on the scientific method. If a patient improved after treatment with a certain herb or plant a doctor would then use this for all the patients he saw with the same symptoms.

Western Medicine slowly became more scientific as tools were developed such as the thermometer, stethoscope, and microscope. As doctors, scientists and others began to cut into dead bodies the structure and function of organs became better understood.

The scientific method slowly came into being offering a framework for the study of nature and the human body. The best research is precise and observes or measures what it wants to study through the most efficient design.

Throughout most of western history medicine has taken one path and science another. Over the last few decades' medicine has begun to put more emphasis on using "evidence based practice." This means a movement from a physician relying solely on what they were taught and what they personally have experienced to using methods to diagnose and treat that have been studied and found beneficial using scientifically designed research involving hundreds, thousands, even tens of thousands of people.

Medicine and health care have been playing catch-up to mainstream science in using the scientific method. It is now trying to establish solid truth about disease, diagnosis and treatment. Areas like cancer (oncology) have been using the scientific method in designing large research for a few decades now and have made great strides in many cancers.

There are gaps in our knowledge about the inner ear leaving Otolaryngology to operate like old time medicine. Sometimes it operates more on a belief system than on careful, welldone research that includes control groups and other methods of getting to the truth. It can still be more about trial and error with each patient.

When done well by trained scientists research is a complicated, expensive and time-consuming process. Because of the difficulty and expense not enough otology research is done to move this area along.

RESEARCH INTO MÉNIÈRE'S

Research into Ménière's disease has been going on for more than a century. Why the lack of substantial progress?

- Diagnosis of Ménière's disease in a living person does not have a "gold standard" test. (A test that can diagnose a disease accurately)

- All the structures inside the inner ear, and their functions, are not fully understood.

- The study of a treatment in a group who may or may not all have the same disorder will not provide accurate results.

The number one priority research area of the NIDCD (within the NIH) is understanding normal function. The second priority area is uderstanding disease and disorders. Researching treatments is in the number three spot in part due to the lack of a gold standard test.

CHAPTER THIRTY-TWO
WHO PAYS FOR RESEARCH?

Research is both intellectually demanding and expensive. Because of the expense, governments provide the lion's share of research funding around the world. In the U.S. it's mostly by the National Institutes of Health, located in Bethesda, Maryland. In Europe funding comes from individual government organizations such as the Medical Research Council of the UK, Inserm in France and from the European Union through the European Research Council. Some other countries providing funding include the National Health and Medical Research Council in Australia, Canadian Institutes of Health Research in Canada, Health Research Council of New Zealand in New Zealand and Japan Agency for Medical Research and Development in Japan.

In the case of medications and devices the money is usually spent by the company developing the drug or device.

NIH
The National Institutes of Health in the U.S. is divided into many different institutes. Each institute has it's own director, budget and areas of study. The institute covering Ménière's disease is the NIDCD, the National Institute on Deafness and other Communication Disorders founded in 1985.

Essentially this institute covers all the body areas an otolaryngologist is responsible for. Hearing, balance, taste, swallowing, the tongue, speech, language, and voice are all in this institutes portfolio. Full information about them can be found at https://www.nidcd.nih.gov

Deafness, by far, receives the most NIDCD funding and balance the least. In fiscal year 2011 hearing received 55%, language 11%, smell 10%, speech 7%, voice 7%, taste 6% and balance 4% of the NIDCD budget. The 2016 budget for the NIH as a whole is approximately $30,000,000,000 (billion) and for the NIDCD approximately $416,000,000 (million). Around 80% of this funding pays for research projects, the rest runs the institute and programs to help train scientists and physicians for careers in research.

What vestibular research is being funded?

- NIDCD spends around $325,000 for the Temporal bone bank located at the Massachusetts Eye and Ear Institute campus in Boston and has done so for at least 2 decades.

- Inner ear fluids research at Washington University, St. Louis since at 1993, $350,000 in fiscal year 2016.

- Research into the autonomic nervous system connections/influence with the vestibular system has been funded for a number of years, $350,000 for fiscal year 2016 at the University of Pittsburg.

- Many pieces of research aimed at delivery of drugs to the inner ear have been funded over the years.

- In fiscal year 2016 over $1,000,000 will be spent on ongoing research into devices to supplement or replace balance including an implantable prosthesis similar to a cochlear implant.

The NIH selects the projects to fund through a competitive process that selects the best research project in a priority area. Research isn't funded just because the money is on hand. Proposed studies must be well designed, doable and usually associated with an experienced primary investigator at a well-established institution with a proven track record. If this doesn't happen the money is not spent.

NIDCD priority areas are:
- Priority Area 1: Understanding Normal Function

- Priority Area 2: Understanding Diseases and Disorders

- Priority Area 3: Improving Diagnosis, Treatment, and Prevention

- Priority Area 4: Improving Outcomes for Human Communication

OTHER AGENCIES

Other U.S. government agencies funding hearing and balance research include the Department of Defense, NASA and National Science Foundation. In the past the DoD was most interested in the prevention and treatment of hearing trauma but now also has a huge interest in traumatic head injury including the symptoms of dizziness and vestibular trauma. NASA has been doing vestibular research for years with a large interest in space sickness. The National Science Foundation funds many different types of research with no specific ear focus.

ORGANIZATIONS

The Ménière's Society of the UK, a patient organization, has helped fund a number of studies and currently has a Smartphone based app project called the Ménière's Monitor, http://www.menieresmonitor.com. Enrolled members in the U.K. grade their symptoms everyday and send the information via the app. The aim is to find out more about the relationship of symptoms to environmental factors. So far there is evidence building for an effect from atmospheric pressure, something known to many with the disorder but not well documented.

COMPANIES

The drug company Otonomy is currently testing a sustained release version of the steroid dexamethasone for transtympanic administration. The study is being conducted in both the U.S. and around Europe. See more about drug studies in the next chapter.

SOME FACTORS MAKING RESEARCH EXPENSIVE

In the US the principle investigator, the person in charge of the research project, is highly educated. Whether they are a PhD, MD or MD/PhD, 8-10 years have been spent in college/university usually racking up impressive student loans currently in the $100,000 to $250,00 range. Not only must their salaries be enough for food, housing, transportation and the other expenses of living, they also need enough money to make payments on their student loans. Universities doing research need to keep the researchers income high enough to keep them away from employment in the private sector as well. Research facilities also tend to be in cities or other places with the highest cost of living.

Depending upon the type research a number of these highly educated professionals are involved as well as others with less advanced degrees. Research can also involve a statistician, computer expert, professional writer, veterinarian, and many other educated/trained individuals.

The work of all these professionals may start months, even years, before the research actually begins. They must work on the research question to be answered and the design of the study that will answer it in the best way. There may also be animal research to determine if the next step into humans can be done.

Equipment, that can be quite expensive, as well as supplies must be purchased and maintained. Computers and special software may be needed. Space for the research must be found and paid for. In human research participants may also be reimbursed for expenses such as travel, food, etc.

The number of people studied, number of locations used and the length of time the study is run all add to the cost.

REFERENCES
https://www.nidcd.nih.gov

CHAPTER THIRTY-THREE
EXPENSE OF DRUG RESEARCH

Drug research is a long and expensive process from idea to approved product. According to the FDA most drugs beginning this process are not approved and the company only spends money with no "payday." Drugs may be shelved because they are not effective, have too many side effects or will not prove profitable for the company.

First, scientists bring the idea to life in the laboratory. If the most basic work looks promising the drug is then tested on animals in a process called pre-clinial trials.

If the pre-clinical trials are favorable the company makes a business decision, not a humanitarian decision, to determine if they should go on. If at any point the drug looks ineffective or does not look profitable a drug company will abandon the work and move on to something else.

When the drug company decides to go forward the drug then undergoes the FDA (Food and drug administration) drug approval process. The application fee alone is approximately $2,000,000 (two million). This pays for the expense of FDA scientists overseeing the process. This money does not pay for the actual process of research, that additional expense is borne by the drug company.

On occasion some of the drug research expense is paid for by a government agency such as the NIH (National Institute of Health) to make sure a drug gets to market. That has been the case in the race toward an Ebola vaccine, for example.

Drug companies are in business to make money, they are not charitable institutions. Their decisions are made to keep the company in business and supply their stockholders with a good return on their investment.

Authors note: I am describing how a drug gets to market, I am not endorsing the method or the profits taken by pharmaceutical companies.

REFERENCES

https://www.fda.gov/forindustry/userfees/prescriptiondruguserfee/
https://www.fda.gov/drugs/resourcesforyou/consumers/ucm143534.htm

CHAPTER THIRTY-FOUR
UNDERSTANDING RESEARCH

Anyone with a background in healthcare science or statistics can read and at least partially understand vestibular and Ménière's disease research published in scientific journals. Without this type background the task becomes very difficult. Time and effort are both needed to understand research.

Each person reading research must be able to evaluate the research to determine its value. Simply being in print does not mean the research has been either designed well or carried out properly. The entire report must be read to make this determination. Reading only the abstract, a summary of the report that is many times available online, is not enough.

What needs to be checked?

- Was the journal peer reviewed, was it read by other leading researchers in the area?

- Have other researchers had similar results?

- Were the number of people studied enough to make a good study?

- Was a control or placebo group used in the study?

Keep in mind that little of Ménière's disease research in print is considered by the "Cochrane Reviews" to be well done and meaningful, usually because the number of people was too small and/or the study lacked a control group

CHAPTER THIRTY-FIVE
PARTICIPATING IN RESEARCH

First, don't participate in research with the goal of improving your own situation in the short term, it most likely won't. Join knowing the information collected may help other people in the future.

In the U.S. the easiest research you can participate in is temporal bone donation. You sign up now to donate your temporal bones at the time of your death. This only requires a bit of paperwork and allowing the temporal bone bank to store a copy of your medical records. Your bones and medical records will be studied in the future to help in understanding vestibular disorders. Ask your specialist about the federally funded temporal bone bank registry or read their webpage at tbregistry.org Once you are signed up there isn't much else to do other than making sure your next of kin will carry this out at the proper time.

To be involved in clinical research right now, speak to your specialist as a starting point. Then check a database for clinical studies, here are a few:

Researchmatch.org
Clinicaltrials.gov
clinicalstudies.info.nih.gov

Recruitment from these webpages is not limited to US citizens and sometimes conducted in overseas locations. Medical research is sometimes conducted by international teams in multiple locations and not always

In the UK check with the Ménière's Society about the research they have underway.

Printed in Great Britain
by Amazon